You Can't Ou~~tsource~~

Weight Loss...

*With a pill or meal delivered to your door.

But You Can Lose Weight and Be Thin Forever

CAPT Ed Boullianne, USN (Ret.)

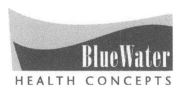

BlueWater
HEALTH CONCEPTS

ISBN number 978-0-9843898-0-3

Library of Congress Control Number: 2010915987

Published by
BlueWater Health Concepts, LLC
Alexandria, VA 22314

www.YouCantOutsourceWeightLoss.com
www.BluewaterHealthConcepts.com

Edited by Ida M. Halasz, Ph.D., Halvan Associates
Cover and Book Design by Karla K. Hills, Art Direction & Graphic Design
Cartoons by Randy Glasbergen (www.glasbergen.com)

Printed in the United States of America

For my Sister
Michelle

"Keep steadily before you the fact that all true success depends at last upon yourself." ~ Theodore T. Hunger

Foreword

On Sunday afternoon August 4th, 2002, I received word that my sister had died. During the call from my brother I asked, "How did this happen?" The short answer was that our older sister Michelle had suffered a massive heart attack while working as a home care nurse with an elderly couple. She had died by the time the paramedics arrived. Dead at the young age of 46, she left behind a husband and 12-year old son.

The longer version of how this happened took me years to discover. Devastated by my sister's death and the effect it had on her extended family, I was determined to discover why so many Americans suffer from obesity and poor health. Knowing what I know now, I would have seen it coming, and hopefully would have been able to help prevent my sister's inevitable downward spiral into obesity and poor health.

My own wake-up call came just two months later. Working as a career officer in the U.S. Navy, I was reviewing the results of my latest annual flight physical with my flight surgeon. Noticing that I had checked the box indicating that a sister or other female relative died before the age of 55, he inquired more closely into my family history. Concerned with my weight, blood pressure and cholesterol readings, he warned me outright, "Take positive steps to improve these numbers, or you will follow your sister into the grave." I was 44 years old.

When the flight surgeon prescribed *Zocor* to lower my cholesterol, he also advised me to improve my overall health and lose some weight, although he didn't tell me exactly how to do it. What followed was an incredible journey of frustration as I tried in desperation to lose weight. Using commercially available programs, I did lose 8-10 pounds, but always gained them back again. This generally occurred with the changing of the seasons, my circumstances at work, or simply because I got tired of doing the things required for losing weight.

> Permanent weight loss is a realistic goal for all of us once we realize that the weight loss process can't be outsourced.

I finally made a breakthrough when I decided, boldly perhaps, that I would figure this "weight loss thing" out for myself. Armed with the Internet, and critical thinking skills honed through years of flying jets for the Navy, I learned the fundamentals of how the human body works. I then used this knowledge to develop my **practices for permanent weight loss.** It was only after I took ownership of the weight loss process that I realized I could be successful. I have shared this information with seminar audiences and have been pleased to hear the results of so many success stories.

This book is the product of all I have learned. Permanent weight loss is a realistic goal for all of us once we realize that the weight loss process can't be outsourced.

About This Book

Although the chapters that follow are the result of what I learned about losing weight, my most important discovery was that **weight loss can't be outsourced!** Little did I know when I made the decision to "figure this weight loss thing out for myself," I would stumble across the key to permanent weight loss. Losing weight is principally a cerebral exercise.

Once I figured out why I was overweight and understood the fundamentals of weight loss, the actual execution of the weight loss process was relatively easy. Yes, easy! I lost 34 pounds in 34 weeks and have kept it off since 2003.

That being said, losing weight is not something you can attempt half-heartedly. While it's okay to be a hacker or Sunday afternoon duffer when it comes to your golf game, you can't approach weight loss in the same manner. Weight loss, especially in today's environment, will require your full attention. Only through education, practice and surrendering some of your old habits, can you be successful.

The Five Basic Truths in Chapter 2 will guide you through the thought process you will need to achieve permanent weight loss. After you complete the self assessment that begins in Chapter 3, you'll be ready to identify and implement those actions, learned skills and practices highlighted in the remaining chapters that will be most effective for your personal weight-loss journey.

> If your goal is permanent weight loss, there's no sense in beginning the process until you understand weight loss in a holistic sense.

The reason that commercial weight-loss programs like *Nutrisystem* don't work is that they leave out these critical first steps. They offer pre-packaged meals or some other gimmicks that don't require any thought. If your goal is permanent weight loss, there's no sense in beginning the process until you understand weight loss in a holistic sense.

Once you complete your self-assessment, you will realize that it's impossible to achieve permanent weight loss with any program that is designed to be executed without having to think. When our car breaks down or our water heater fails, we call someone to fix it. We may not care why it failed, but inevitably ask, "How much is the repair going to cost, and how quickly can it be fixed?" If this has been your approach to weight loss, the concepts in this book will be liberating, and you too will claim it was "easy."

Many people in my seminars tell me that they really do want a program that doesn't require them to think. Pop the meals in the microwave, eat what they send you, and lose weight. If you stick with their meal program at $300 - $700 a month, you'll probably lose some weight, but when the meals stop coming, then what? What's the plan when you go out to eat, or get invited to a dinner party or barbeque? You're on your own without having learned the critical skills for maintaining the weight loss you've achieved.

> Weight loss requires education, incentive and practice.

Don't be fooled by the commercial weight loss world's advertising. Well-paid and incentivized celebrities claim how easy it was to lose 20, 30 and even 40 pounds. Just "pop the meals into the microwave" they tell us and magically the weight will just melt right off. Don't forget to read the fine print though, where they are legally bound to state, **"weight loss not typical."**

The strategy of weight loss organizations is to trot out a widely known celebrity to make you believe that you can effortlessly lose weight just as they did. The only difference is that you have a real job and you are not getting paid a half million dollars for your weight loss. Weight loss requires education, incentive and practice.

Call *Nutrisystem* and ask them what exactly "results not typical" means. The cold hard fact is that the vast majority of us have absolutely nothing to show for the billions we collectively spend on these weight-loss schemes. Programs like *Nutrisystem* are financially successful for stockholders ($61 million in profit for nearly three quarters of a billion in sales for 2008) but they deliver abysmal results for the individuals trying to lose weight. If any of these programs really worked, wouldn't we all be skinny?

Additionally, don't ever buy any of those magical weight loss pills you see advertised on the Internet. If there really were a pill that worked for weight loss, permanent or otherwise, wouldn't the pharmaceutical companies provide it to us via our prescription drug plans? Clearly, pills are not the way to approach successful and permanent weight loss.

Yes, there is quite a bit to assimilate, and some of the information will be more important for you than others. Your self-assessment will also help you in choosing the five most effective tools to populate your own "Guiding Star" in the final chapter.

This book has the information and tools you need to lose weight and keep it off forever. It will help you develop an inquisitive, questioning mind when it comes to nutrition and weight-loss information. You'll never fall for any of those quick weight loss schemes after you read this book. I promise that if you use the tools in this book to navigate your way through a personal weight loss journey, you can lose weight and keep it off, <u>forever</u>.

Your guide to a healthier life,

Ed Boullianne

Contents

Charts and Illustrations

1

The Facts

Two-thirds of Americans today are either overweight or obese. Obesity-related health care costs American employers an unbelievable 147 billion dollars a year.

The cost in lost productivity in the workplace is mounting and is more than the cost associated with tobacco use. A skilled or knowledge worker with a Body Mass Index (BMI) of 27 or higher can cost a company $10,000 per year in weight-related absenteeism. That's just the cost of not showing up for work. For perspective, an individual who is 5'6" tall and weighs 170 pounds has a BMI of 27, the same as someone 5'10" tall that weighs 190 pounds.

Health-related medical costs are even more astronomical. David Rebich* at the Department of Treasury states that the US Government would have to set aside $38 trillion dollars today just to cover the shortfall in Medicare over the next 75 years. Annual total Medicare costs are running more than $600 billion dollars a year, exceeded only by Social Security and defense outlays. Total US medical costs for 2009 were $2.5 trillion, or more than $8,000 per person. This is before we start to incur the additional costs of the newly legislated health care reform.

In the June 2007 issue of *Money Magazine*, the editor's note had two salient points. First, it quoted Paul Fronstin

*Email to Ed Boullianne, 5-24-2010 from David Rebich, the Assistant Commissioner for Government-wide Accounting at the Financial Management Service (US Treasury) who prepares the government's monthly budget report and annual Financial Statement stated that the "Present Value of the 75-year Actuarial Projections for Medicare (Parts A, B, and D) costs will be approximately $38 trillion." In other words, this is the present value of the current unfunded obligations under Medicare (all parts), and we would have to set aside $38 trillion dollars today to cover the principal and interest for the shortfall over the next 75 years.

of the Employee Benefit Research Institute who stated, "A 65 year-old couple could need savings of $295,000 just to cover insurance premiums and out-of-pocket medical costs." How many of us have that much saved just to cover our health care? Additionally, the editor Eric Schurenberg recommended that it would be "Smarter to lead your life so that you need less health care in the first place." That is great advice for us Americans as we get fatter by the day.

With today's modern medicine and emergency care, most of us have the ability to live into old age. Unless you are one of the unfortunate few to die traumatically (car crash, hit by lightening, etc.), you <u>will</u> more than likely die of cancer, heart disease or stroke. Therefore, it seems to me that we should all use preventive strategies to delay the onset of these diseases and to maintain our quality of life.

The strategy I'm proposing is very simple! The number one thing we can do to improve our health and lower our health care costs is to achieve an "appropriate weight for our height." Not smoking, or using tobacco products, is a very close number two. The problem is that most of us don't know how to lose weight. Many of us also have a skewed perspective of what is a normal, appropriate weight for good health. Sadly, the commercially available weight loss programs fail to educate us on how to achieve and maintain an appropriate weight for our height.

> The number one thing we can do to improve our health and lower our health care costs is to achieve an "appropriate weight for our height."

This book is not about losing weight fast and makes no claims about amazing results. It <u>doesn't</u> recommend a deprivation or gimmicky diet, or actions that require super-human willpower. It <u>does</u> provide the facts about how the human body works, its limitations, and the information needed to effect realistic and <u>permanent</u> weight loss. This book also recognizes that we are all different, so it doesn't assume that "one size fits all." It puts you in charge, based on the skills and information you acquire to manage your own weight for the rest of your life.

Finally, losing weight isn't just about how you'll look, although you'll more than likely look better and feel more confident about your appearance. It's about the quality of your life, preventing disease, increasing longevity, not spending your money on medical expenses, and saving national health care dollars*. It's also about something that is rarely mentioned—providing a role model and teaching critical life skills to our children.

*In an interview on CNBC with Erin Burnett on November 4th 2010, legendary hedge fund manager and Tiger Management Chairman Julian Robertson stated that if we could return to 1991's obesity rates in the US it would "add $ 1 Trillion to the GDP."

2

Five Basic Truths

During my weight loss journey, I discovered five basic truths that are essential to sustained and permanent weight loss. Understanding these truths is vital before you begin your weight loss journey. They'll make sense whether or not you previously tried to lose weight. They are:

Basic Truth #1: If you're tired, hungry, or craving foods, you won't lose weight.

There is no way you can sustain a weight loss journey (seven months in my case), if you don't learn how to do it without being tired, hungry, and craving your favorite foods all the time. If you are constantly hungry, or have no energy during a weight loss journey, then your body is telling you you're not doing it right. The key to successful weight loss is to discover how to still enjoy eating, while simultaneously losing weight.

Basic Truth #2: Only make lifestyle or diet changes that you can maintain forever.

The reason most diets don't work is because they require you to make drastic, unrealistic and unsustainable changes to your diet or lifestyle. Yes, the science behind many of the commercial weight loss programs is reasonably sound, and you may lose weight, but only as long as you strictly adhere to them. The problem is that they're nearly impossible to stick with, and even if you do, what have you learned when you're done? Nothing! Most people go right back to living and eating as they did previously, and invariably regain the weight.

> Permanent weight loss only comes with permanent changes.

Permanent weight loss only comes with permanent changes. Outsourcing your weight loss to a pill or meal delivered to your door will never alter your diet and lifestyle long enough or sufficiently enough to produce permanent results. Figuring out the changes you're willing to make—hopefully forever—requires a lot of thought, a little practice and some trial and error*. I traded the unhealthy foods that I discovered were not good for me for healthier ones that I really enjoyed eating.

> Figuring out the changes you're willing to make—hopefully forever— requires a lot of thought, a little practice and some trial and error.

That being said, I must confess that I flatly refused to give up pepperoni pizza and red wine because I was not willing to give them up forever. But I lost weight because I stuck to the key principles in this book. You too can lose weight without depriving yourself of everything you love to eat and drink!

Basic Truth #3: Listen to your body.

We potty train our children by teaching them to "listen to their bodies" and then immediately begin a lifelong program teaching them to ignore it. Have you ever had your children say, "I'm not hungry anymore," only to tell them to finish everything on their plate? How many of us eat for emotional reasons instead of in response to true hunger? Add that to the constant communication we receive from this hyper-connected world that tells us to eat, drink or buy the latest product Madison Avenue is hawking. Our children and young adults are their latest target audiences, and not surprisingly, are the fastest growing groups of overweight Americans.

> You too can lose weight without depriving yourself of everything you love to eat and drink!

As you slowly start to make changes in your diet and lifestyle, your body will tell you if you're getting it right and if

---

* Trial and error: The willingness to try new ideas, foods, drink choices, exercise regimens, etc in order to discover what works best for your weight loss journey.

you'll be able to do it forever. The best way to start is to ask, "Why am I eating this?" Are you eating because you're hungry and need to refuel the tank? Or are you eating just because it feels good, there's food available in a social setting, you're bored, angry, celebrating or trying to fill an emotional void in your life? When we re-learn how to listen and understand what our bodies tell us, we begin to know when we are eating for the wrong reasons.

Basic Truth #4: Willpower and deprivation are not weight-loss tools.

We humans are so bad at self-denial that it surprises me when I see diets that are based on deprivation and the exercise of super-human willpower. Once you've learned the fundamentals of weight loss, you'll never ever consider subjecting yourself to one of those diets, or even trying to use willpower or deprivation to lose weight. Self-discipline and educating yourself on the basics of nutrition and how the human body realistically works, on the other hand, are very effective weight loss tools.

Basic Truth #5: The human body was meant to move.

Oh, you just knew I was going to mention exercise. While the good news is that you don't have to run for hours on a treadmill, you can't just sit in front of that computer screen all day when you're trying to achieve a healthy weight.

The human body loses weight and functions best when it is involved in some level of exertion. Think **brisk walking** or taking the stairs instead of the elevator at work. Playing ball with the kids, gardening, and yes, even cleaning the house can all count as exercise. Studies show that <u>most</u> people who lose weight engage in moderate exercise on a regular basis. While many of us feel we could happily exist without any exercise in our lives, the reality is that without some exercise we can't achieve a healthy weight and long-term quality of life.

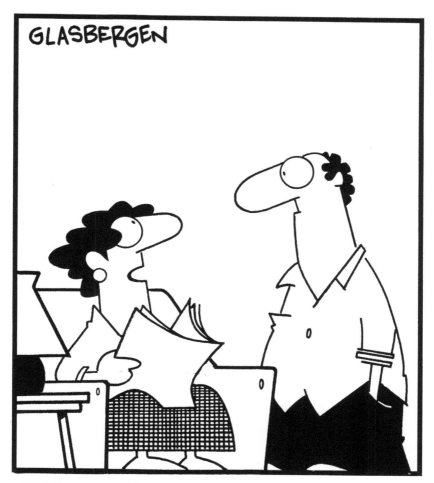

"This magazine says we can lose 25 pounds in a week by eating chocolate cake 3 times a day. Finally, a diet that makes sense!"

3

Self-Assessment

In my attempt to figure out weight loss, I dissected my potential reasons for being overweight into four basic categories. I realized that together—

"What" foods I ate,

"Why" I ate them,

"How Much Food" I ate and

"How Much I Moved"

determined what I weighed. Only by conducting a "self-assessment" of each these categories did I discover where I needed to focus my weight loss efforts.

A self-assessment will help you determine which of these four categories is mostly responsible for your overweight condition. A self-assessment will also help you to re-learn to listen to your body (Basic Truth # 3).

In my case I bought a small pocket-sized spiral notebook (a log book as we call it in the Navy), to record each of the four categories every day. I'd read about this somewhere and didn't initially consider it until I realized I couldn't remember what I ate for lunch two days ago. Each day I recorded what and how much food I ate, how it made me feel, the time I ate it, the reason I ate it and how much I moved or exercised*.

This was a typical day for me BEFORE my weight loss journey:

---

*Fill-in Meal Logs are provided on Pages 172-174 for your use.

Date/ Time	What + how much food I ate	Why I ate these	How I felt	How much I moved
4-11 Breakfast	Bagel w/ cream cheese = 436 calories, tall latte = 336	Quick, easy to eat in car; stopped for latte at favorite coffee shop	Woke me up, still a little hungry	Drove car to the office
4-11 Lunch	Big Mac = 540 calories, fries = 380, med. Coke = 210	Busy day, had to have fast food lunch	Full and a little sleepy	Treadmill 5 miles in office gym before lunch
4-11 Dinner	3 slices pepperoni pizza = 720 calories, tossed salad = 33 + dressing = 70, 2+ glasses red wine = 260	It's Friday night and I always have pizza and wine on Friday night	Could have eaten more but stopped myself	Played catch with my older son for 45 min before dinner
Total	2985 calories			

Keeping the log took some effort, but it turned out to be an extremely valuable and important exercise. It took me about 10 days to discover that it was "What" I ate that was largely responsible for my weight gain. It was easy to gain weight with some of these foods filled with calories, fat, sodium and sugar. The information on the chart above indicated I was 985 calories above the healthy 2000 recommended daily calories*.

I learned that I ate three times a day and didn't snack much between meals. For the most part, I didn't appear to eat in response to emotional needs. Although I must confess that in the months that followed, I realized that I ate nearly an entire pizza when I was tired or angry.

We are all different. You may say that I had it easy because I simply had to change what I ate instead of getting used to a workout routine or handling the more complex issues of emotional eating. That could be so, but to change the "What," I had to learn much more about the right foods to eat for weight loss.

> Keeping the log took some effort, but it turned out to be an extremely valuable and important exercise.

---

* I never actually counted or recorded the calories in my food log (journal). Calories are provided just to illustrate that "What" eaters consume more calories than they burn because of the food choices they make.

I've met people who ate the right foods and were not emotional eaters. When they started a moderate exercise regimen, the weight just melted away. Was it easier for them? Possibly, but I don't think so. They were successful because they focused their efforts on the areas of their lives that were out of balance.

I'll note here that as a Naval Flight Officer, I lived in a culture of physical fitness and ran five miles a day, yet I was still overweight. One of my first discoveries was that exercise was not the key to weight loss, at least not for me. Using the self-assessment process, I discovered that I needed to make changes in other areas of my life, mostly in the types of foods I ate.

> Again, we are all different, and only by examining our own personal habits can we begin to discover where we need to focus our weight loss efforts.

Again, we are all different, and only by examining our own personal habits can we begin to discover where we need to focus our weight loss efforts. I can't emphasize enough the importance of completing your self-assessment.

I've read about people who've had their stomachs stapled to prevent them from chronic overeating. They later discovered that their issue was a deeply rooted emotional problem that manifested itself in another addictive behavior such as alcohol or drug abuse. Their life-threatening surgery addressed the symptom, not the underlying cause. Some of them, unable to overeat, resorted to even more self-destructive behaviors. There are clearly less dangerous and more effective ways to approach permanent weight loss.

4
"What" Eaters

In general, "**What**" eaters need to change the types of food they eat. The Food Stoplight Chart, Calorie Guide to the Most Popular Drinks, and the chapter on calorie density should help if you identify this as an area of focus for you. Remember, the key is to still enjoy food. Never eat something you don't like just because it will help you lose weight. You can't put up with that for the rest of your life, can you?

That being said, **do** try foods that you think you don't like. If you haven't had Brussels sprouts since you were 11 years old, try them

> Remember, the key is to still enjoy food.

again. In fact, I recommend that you try them, or any new food, at least three times. If you can still honestly say you don't like the taste or texture of a food after three attempts, cross it off your list. There are many other healthy choices.

I found I began to crave foods that I previously thought I disliked. The key was that I was able to substitute healthy, low calorie foods that I enjoyed for foods that were less healthy and loaded with calories. I still enjoyed eating, so the changes in my diet were not really difficult to maintain. The key for me was <u>planning</u>. I ate breakfast at home and brought my lunch to work each day. This way I knew I'd have something to eat that I liked, which is a key to success for most of us.

By training myself to eat the right foods day-to-day, I was better prepared when I was invited to one of those high calorie feasts we call dinner parties. Today I can confidently navigate my way around the buffet table and make better choices. I now automatically think before I dive into a dish that has too many calories for the short-lived fun it provides.

Dr. Steven Pratt M.D., the author of two excellent books (*Superfoods Rx* and *Superfoods Healthstyle*) identified 24 "*superfoods*" as dramatically better for our health and longevity than other foods. I added these *superfoods* into my diet and was amazed how well my body responded. I had more energy and found, surprisingly, that I really enjoyed them. The best part was that I was also losing weight!

I've highlighted the 24 *superfoods* on the **Food Stoplight Chart** in Chapter 20 and it's there that you'll find a complete list of the plant based foods you should be eating (Green Light), and those that are calorie dense that you should eat sparingly (Red Light). No matter what your results are from the self-assessment, you should try to add these *superfoods* to your diet. Your body really needs the natural, plant based foods Dr. Pratt recommends instead of the processed fare that is so readily available these days.

Our bodies thrive when we eat plant based foods, but we also have to understand that we are pre-programmed to seek and eat calorie-dense foods such as cheeseburgers and steak. To survive, especially when food has been difficult to acquire, human beings have always sought the most calorie-dense foods. Today, we need to realize that there are far more calorie-dense foods available than we need for our relatively sedentary lifestyles.

Your Focus Areas as a "What" Eater:

1. Choose natural, plant based foods that are low in calorie density such as carrots, cantaloupe and whole grain bread. Since many beverages are very high in calories, making better drink choices is a key element in losing weight for "What" eaters.

2. Visualize what those high fat and calorie-laden foods are doing to your health. It became much easier to select healthier food when I connected my poor food choices to my elevated blood pressure and cholesterol readings.

3. Plan your meals and buy the food in advance for lunches and other meals away from home unless you know that healthy food will be available. Meal planning is essential, especially during a busy work week. Don't let the office vending machine or local fast food restaurant decide what you'll eat.

> Meal planning is essential, especially during a busy work week.

4. Exercise and sleep are key elements for most "What" eaters. When you exercise, you burn calories, especially those in the fun foods you want (such as my pepperoni pizza). Sleep regulates your hormone levels and helps curb those cravings for high calorie-dense foods.

5. Reward yourself occasionally with foods that won't torpedo a week's worth of healthy eating. Taking a night off from your weight loss program can really help keep you going for the long haul. Think, "pizza and wine, Friday night." Once you're at your target weight you can use a five-day on, two-day off approach. I'm very careful about what I eat Monday through Friday, and then "cheat," **a little**, on the weekends.

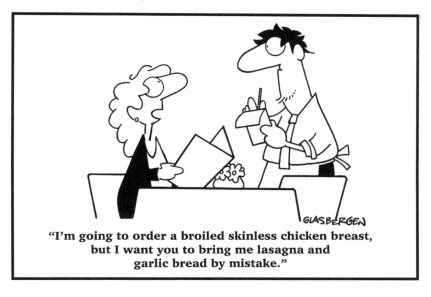

"I'm going to order a broiled skinless chicken breast, but I want you to bring me lasagna and garlic bread by mistake."

5
"Why" Eaters

"Why" eaters run the gamut. A year after a young woman attended one of my seminars, she told me that my talk "changed her life." When I asked how, she said she started to look at food in an entirely different light. She used the self-assessment and correctly identified herself as a "Why" eater. Soon afterwards, she began questioning everything she ate, not so much whether it was the right food, but if she was eating it for the **right reasons**. In short, she began eating in response to true hunger and stopped using food in response to boredom or other normal emotional needs.

During a year of intensive study for her Master's degree, she used the insight from her self-assessment to lose 30 pounds. She's kept them off and feels great. And yes, she looks great too! It's important to note that she probably eats many of the higher calorie density foods that I as a "What" eater, generally avoid.

"Why" eaters get their extra calories from eating for the wrong reasons, while "What" eaters, like me, get too many calories from eating the wrong foods. Unlike "What" eaters, it's not so much the right foods that count, but eating them for the right reasons. Don't get me wrong, good nutrition counts. It just counts more for some of us than for others! Many "Why" eaters discover that they can eat almost anything, within reason, when they learn to eat only in response to true hunger. It sure doesn't seem fair, especially to us "What" eaters, but that's the way it is.

While as a "What" eater I had to train myself to make better food choices, "Why" eaters need to develop the skills to eat in response to true hunger. At parties, "Why" eaters need to ensure they are not eating just because there is food available, while I need to ensure that I'm making the right food choices. I don't generally eat for emotional reasons, so when I'm full, I stop eating. If I choose the right foods, my calorie intake is more in line with the calories I burn each day.

> "Why" eaters need to ensure they are not eating just because there is food available.

"Why" eaters can, at times, continue to eat even after they are full or eat again before they are truly hungry. Many "Why" eaters unfortunately have learned how well food seems to address their emotional issues. When "Why" eaters learn to eat for the right reasons, it's not just the choice of food that keep their calories in line, but the choice not to eat in the first place.

Do you see how two different people, both on weight loss journeys, need to approach the same social gathering scenario with different strategies? This is why doing the self-assessment and learning the Five Basic Truths (Chapter 2) are such vital first steps when trying to achieve permanent weight loss, and why so many commercial weight loss programs fail.

Unfortunately, not all "Why" eaters are like the young woman described above. In spite of correctly identifying themselves as "Why" eaters, some people have deeply-rooted emotional issues and have learned to use food to try to help themselves feel better, or to fuel self-destructive behavior. Many have been overweight since childhood and carry the baggage of low self-esteem and question their self-worth.

> Some people have deeply-rooted emotional issues and have learned to use food to try to help themselves feel better, or to fuel self-destructive behavior.

For this type of "Why" eater, weight loss is almost entirely a mental process. These eaters must first learn to change how they think about themselves. In many cases, it is the realization that they have been using food as a substitute for self-help that begins the weight loss process. When the "Why" eaters realize why they are overeating, they may start to look at food entirely differently. Those chocolate chip cookies or that cheesecake in the refrigerator may no longer have a vice-grip hold on them. Sure, they still may have a cookie or two, but they won't eat the entire box any longer. "Why" eaters make real progress when they refuse to let that person staring back at them in the mirror make them believe that they are unworthy of happiness and good health.

> We are all different, and one single weight loss approach, while successful for many of us, won't work for all of us.

We are all different, and one single weight loss approach, while successful for many of us, won't work for all of us. This is my biggest complaint about the weight loss world and is one of the reasons for writing this book. I believe that the "one size fits all" approach is actually counterproductive. When we read the testimonials from people who have had great success with a certain weight loss approach, and then fail to get the same results, we are understandably discouraged.

This book is for all types of eaters because it begins with a self-assessment that helps you discover where you are out of balance. Until you discover that, I can't help to "make you thin."

> This book is for all types of eaters because it begins with a self-assessment that helps you discover where you are out of balance.

There are several major problems with programs like *Nutrisystem*, *Jenny Craig* and *Diet to Go*. First, they can't deliver permanent weight loss for "Why" eaters, a vast majority of their female client base, because their diets are based on portion control and lowering calorie density. "Why" eaters must learn to eat for the right reasons, generally by figuring out what emotional "triggers" (depression, boredom, anger, stress, etc.) lead them to eat for the wrong reasons.

Following a pre-set, portion-controlled commercial diet

program that is designed so that "you don't have to think" is exactly the opposite of what "Why" eaters need to do. Sure, "Why" eaters can lose weight on these plans, but only temporarily. When their meals stop arriving, they are left without having developed the learned responses, or behaviors, that will help them avoid eating for the wrong reasons.

Second, these programs don't teach the "What" and "How Much" eaters anything, nor prepare them for the realities of the real world. They don't teach you how to cook their very low calorie density lasagna that helped you lose weight.

Third, what's the plan when the meals stop coming? Most people who buy these programs go right back to their old eating habits and lifestyle without having learned how to function in the real world and invariably gain back the weight they lost.

Fourth, unless you're a hermit with deep pockets who stays at home all the time, you'll find it impossible to continue the meal plans indefinitely. If you don't go broke paying for meals and shipping costs, you'll quickly realize that meals delivered to your door don't really fit your busy lifestyle. Watching your kids play baseball at the ballpark until 8:00 PM (smelling those grilled burgers) will relegate those prepared dinners to the back of the cupboard.

> These weight loss plans are just trying to get you to eat fewer calories of the same types of foods that got you into trouble in the first place.

Last of all, the commercial weight loss programs are all based on eating their version of lasagna, pizza, burgers and chocolate. When you get right down to it, these weight loss plans are just trying to get you to eat fewer calories of the same types of foods that got you into trouble in the first place. Most of us must realize that we need to eat better quality, more nutritious food and steer away from the comfort, junk and nutritionally poor choices that have become so much a part of the typical American diet.

> Commercial weight loss companies provide exactly what we think we want: a way to outsource our weight loss so we don't have to think about it.

If you're an *ESPN* fan like I am, you may have noticed that during the commercial breaks, the first ad is for the latest cheese stuffed crust pizza, followed by a commercial for *Nutrisystem*. Isn't this crazy? One product makes you fat, the other promises to make you lose weight, yet they're all selling the same types of food. This is the world you live in!

However, we really can't place all of the blame on the commercial weight loss companies. They provide exactly what we think we want: a way to outsource our weight loss so we don't have to think about it. The only problem is that these programs don't deliver permanent weight loss. As I stated earlier, we have very little to show for the billions we collectively spend on them. That's why we must do a self-assessment and then use our new knowledge to both lose weight and maintain it in the real world.

Remember, if any of these weight loss programs really worked, we'd all be skinny. Ask anyone who has lost weight and kept it off for a year or more how they did it. I mean really discuss how they did it! It won't take too many individual discussions to realize that each of them discovered where they were "out of balance" and then engaged in realistic strategies to implement permanent changes.

One final note: My wife believes that many people simply use programs like *Diet to Go* as their personal chef, or as a fast food option so they don't have to think about what to eat or spend much time preparing meals. I agree this may be a more nutritious choice than other fast food options, but the wrong option if their goal is permanent weight loss.

> If any of these weight loss programs really worked, we'd all be skinny.

You Can't Outsource Weight Loss... But You Can Lose Weight and Be Thin Forever!

Your Focus Areas as a "Why" Eater:

1. Ask yourself, "Why am I eating this?" Be honest with yourself. If you're following Basic Truth #3, you'll start to develop the skills to identify those triggers that cause you to eat in response to emotional needs (see the next chapter for more information on how to do this). Learn to eat in response to true hunger, not to fuel emotional needs or prolong self-destructive behavior.

2. Eat slowly, chew your food completely, and learn to enjoy the taste of your food. As I tell my seminar audiences, "savor the flavor." Why eaters need to be "present in the moment," to focus on what they are eating and avoid the tendency to just shovel the food in their mouth.

3. Learn to recognize when you are full and then stop eating. Physically removing yourself from the table or the room with the food can really help. Don't watch TV while eating and *Tivo* your favorite shows so you're not subjected to all those food commercials after dinner.

4. Willpower, as you now know, is not a weight loss tool. If you're craving chocolate, have a piece…one piece, then walk away. You won't believe how liberating this simple act can be.

5. Exercise is generally not a key tactic for many "Why" eaters, but Basic Truth #5 says we all need to program movement into our sedentary lifestyles. You'll feel great if you exercise enough to get the blood pumping and be amazed at how confident it will make you feel.

6. Getting enough sleep is important for keeping your hormone levels in balance so you'll have a fighting chance with those food cravings.

7. Portion control is often recommended for emotional or "Why" eaters, but I believe it's counterproductive. It's too close to the commercial weight loss programs' tactics so I don't advocate it except perhaps at the very beginning of a weight loss journey for a "Why" eater. It's only when you can break that connection between your eating habits and emotions that you'll be successful.

6

I'm a "Why" or Emotional Eater, so What Can I Do About It?

If you've identified yourself as a "Why" eater, you're to be congratulated for successfully completing the Self-Assessment Process. "Why," or emotional eating, is no doubt responsible for a large portion of this country's overweight population. I've read estimates that claim up to 75 percent of overweight individuals fall into this category.

The good news is that if you've identified yourself as a person that eats for reasons other than true hunger, you can begin the process to change your habits. The bad news is that, depending on where you fall on the scale of emotional eating, you can be the hardest to "fix." Don't despair; this chapter is just for you.

> Emotional eating, is no doubt responsible for a large portion of this country's overweight population.

First, let's review the classic indicators of emotional eating.

✓ **Do you...**

❑ Eat even when you realize that you're not really hungry?

❑ Use food to address anger, loneliness, sadness, stress or pressure at work?

❑ Eat because you're bored, frustrated or anxious?

❑ Eat when you're concerned about relationship issues?

❑ Eat alone (by choice) or try to hide that you are eating?

❑ Feel guilty about your eating?

✓ **Do you...**

❑ Eat until you feel miserable or sick?

❑ Feel you have no control over your eating habits?

❑ Find that you gravitate towards situations with large amounts of food where you can overindulge?

❑ Find that your eating is tied to certain situations (watching TV, going to sporting event, movies, etc.), is related to certain smells (burgers grilling, cookies baking) or triggered by visual cues (TV commercials, billboard advertising, etc.)?

If you can check two or more of these indicators you **may** be a "Why" or emotional eater. You also may have an eating disorder, which is more serious. There are two other resources that can help you know for sure. The first is the *Eating Attitudes Test* or the *EAT-26*, the second is the *SCOFF Eating Disorder Quiz*, both available online (use *Google* to find the latest versions).

The reason I mention both is because it is important to know if you are a garden variety emotional eater or if you have an eating disorder that may require professional help. You may benefit from using one of these self-administered programs to identify the reasons, or the "triggers" that cause you to overeat. Then you can learn to do something else besides eat when they occur.

It won't be easy, at least not at first, to make these changes. However, you're already way ahead of the game as you're not wasting your time and money (as my sister did) on meals delivered to your door. Those, as you know, have a zero chance of helping you work through your issues and achieving permanent weight loss.

The first thing I usually tell emotional eaters is that I'd like to take them out into the woods for a few days and let them get lost. They think I'm a madman until I explain that this is a great way for emotional eaters to experience true hunger. Most emotional eaters have not experienced how true hunger feels because they eat so often their bodies have not had to send them the physiological signals in a very long time.

> Don't beat yourself up if you realize that you've eaten for emotional reasons, but do make a note of which trigger(s) caused you to backslide.

Your first exercise is to force yourself to do without food for a good portion of a day. Pick a weekend day so that it doesn't affect your work performance. Second, plan a busy day that includes lots of physical activity. For example, have just a cup of coffee or tea first thing in the morning and then clean the house from top to bottom. Depending on when you started, it should be sometime between mid-morning and early afternoon by the time you begin to feel the physiological signals of true hunger. If you feel light-headed or woozy, you're really hungry and it's time to eat.

Over the next weeks and months you'll need to reinforce feeling true hunger and to acknowledge when you fall back into your old habit of eating before true hunger sets in. Don't beat yourself up if you realize that you've eaten for emotional reasons, but do make a note of which trigger(s) caused you to backslide. It may be time to get out that logbook and write a few notes so that you don't repeat the same mistakes over and over again.

Don't allow yourself to feel guilt and depressed for the inevitable mistakes along the way. I've noticed that when men fall off the weight loss wagon they say, "I screwed up" and move on without having negative feelings about themselves. Women, on the other hand, seem to beat themselves up mercilessly and allow the same anger, guilt and frustration that caused them to eat in the first place to come full circle when they mess up. Don't allow this to happen to you.

> Don't allow yourself to feel guilt and depressed for the inevitable mistakes along the way.

The next thing an emotional eater needs to do is figure out how to replace eating when they experience any of the 10 triggers listed previously. The goal is to find a positive outlet that nurtures your mind, body and soul. Although I'm primarily a "What" eater, when I feel down or stressed out, I go to the gym. I'd rather beat the daylights out of those expensive machines than beat myself up.

You may already be aware of the distractions that work for you. I've heard of dozens of things that emotional eaters do, such as gardening, cleaning the house, taking a walk, crafting, taking a bubble bath, engaging the kids in a one-on-one basketball game, reading, playing sports, playing Solitaire and so forth.

If you can say, "Okay, I'm stressed out, bored or angry and usually I'd go and eat something, but now I'm going to go for a walk instead," you've made progress. Not only did you not consume some calorie-dense junk food, but you got a little exercise to boot! Even if you're only doing this a few times a week, you're making progress. Those calories you didn't eat go into the weight loss bank account. Like our systematic savings programs, it's amazing how quickly a few calories here and there add up to sustained weight loss.

Another method that works for some emotional eaters is to force themselves to wait 20-30 minutes before reaching for something to eat. Emotional eaters tell me that in the rare circumstances when they simply don't have access to food, the craving for food passes within a half hour or so. There aren't many situations anymore when food isn't available, so this "timeout" period is a good skill to develop.

Unfortunately, not everyone is as successful as the young woman in Chapter 5 who quickly worked herself through the self-assessment process to ultimately lose 30 pounds. Some "Why" eaters have such deep-rooted emotional issues that overeating is just the tip of the iceberg when it comes to the problems they have. If you understand the connection between your emotions and the triggers that prompt you to eat, yet you can't actually replace positive activities for binge eating, then you may fall into one of the following categories:

The Mommy Syndrome – From what I have seen, this label applies to smart women who easily understand the principles outlined above (and in this book) but never seem to find the time to implement them. They are generally busy working moms, but can also be professionals dedicated to their work. Somewhere in these women's DNA is a code that says they have to address and meet everyone's needs before their own. With today's busy lifestyles, it's easy to never find time to care for themselves. These women stoically wear the battle scars of their devotion to immediate and extended family and work, without realizing that what the people in their lives really want is a wife, mother or daughter to devote some time to their own happiness and well-being.

I've seen many mothers who fall into this category learn to flip the switch and say, "the next hour is mommy time." They learn that taking care of themselves is just as important as taking care of everyone else. Dads can learn to help by picking up a few "mom" duties so that their spouses can go to the gym or just sit quietly and read. I cook dinner a couple of times a week so my wife can hit the gym on the way home from work, or just relax in the bath tub before our family meal.

The Relationship from Hell – I've seen many people in bad relationships who seek solace in food. These overeaters really don't want that half gallon of ice cream. They'd rather have someone they can talk to and explain the emotions they are feeling. They seem to benefit most from group counseling, because when they have an outlet for their emotions through the discussions, they find that they don't need the comfort of junk food any longer.

While most emotional eaters in this category seem to have bad relationships with their significant other, some have relationships from hell with a bad boss, co-worker, or other dysfunctional family members. It's only when an emotional eater in this category addresses the root cause that they can stop overeating. That may mean getting out of a bad relationship, finding a new job, or distancing themselves from dysfunctional family members.

The Addict – Just as we can't tell drug addicts or alcoholics that they should just stop taking drugs / alcohol to alleviate their problems, we can't tell emotional eaters to just stop eating. These emotional eaters may know they shouldn't use food to address their emotional problems, but they just can't seem to stop. I'm not a doctor or a psychiatrist, but I'm convinced these people use food to fuel self-destructive behavior. For these addicts, instead of using drugs or alcohol, their weapon of individual self-destruction just happens to be food.

There's help for virtually every "Why" eater out there, but some may need to realize that their journey is not going to move directly to the uplifting, positive journey that many of the other types of eaters experience. I have met and spoken with recovered emotional eaters that had to go through a gut-wrenching experience of discovering the demons in their lives. Many of the issues they had to work through began in childhood and resulted from very strained and difficult parental relationships and / or experiences in early adulthood. Yes, this will be a difficult process to undertake, but the result can be the release from a life enslaved to food.

It's not a good marketing technique in a weight loss book to tell the truth, nor explain that implementing the principles will be very difficult for some people. Nonetheless, all of the recommendations in this book can help you achieve permanent weight loss, but only when you're mentally ready to do so.

If you just can't stop eating for emotional reasons, consider enlisting the help of a professional counselor to better prepare you mentally to succeed.

All of the recommendations in this book can help you achieve permanent weight loss, but only when you're mentally ready to do so.

7

"How Much" Eaters

"How Much" eaters are the ones that benefit most from the commercial weight loss programs. They simply eat too much. These programs provide meals that are portion-controlled and low in calories. Their meals attempt to align the amount of food (calories) eaten each day with the calories that are burned. The only problem is that someone else is making the choices for these "How Much" eaters, and they'll have to stick with the program for it to work.

So what happens when a "How Much" eater is invited to someone's house for a dinner party? Do they show up with a weight loss program prepared meal and ask the host to pop it in the microwave for them? Or, what do they do if they're still hungry after they finish the prepared meal?

In many cases, "How Much" eaters have generally learned how good food makes them feel, so they just eat too much. In my seminars with adults, I compare food to sex. In *Letterman* fashion I count down a list and identify the reasons food is better than sex. People always laugh when I say, "We don't have to eat the same food every day." But the top reason, especially for over-50 guys like me, is that "I can eat three times a day!" Sure it gets great laughs, but it also makes a good point.

> "How Much" eaters have generally learned how good food makes them feel, so they just eat too much.

We humans were designed to derive great pleasure from eating and sex, so our early ancestors wouldn't forget to do either one. Life was hard for them and survival of the human species required that we stayed focused on eating and procreation. We still have these same focuses.

It's just that food, in all its amazing varieties and availability, is much easier to get than sex. Well, at least for some of us! Seriously, even I as a "What" eater realized that once I started to give food the same respect as sex, and learned to enjoy it within similar bounds, my relationship with food and my weight both improved.

I also discovered that many "How Much" eaters have become addicted to the salt, sugar and fats that are so prevalent in our food. The American food industry understands this all too well, and has designed foods around these three deadly, and addictive, ingredients. Unfortunately, about 25 percent of Americans never "habituate" to these ingredients according to David Kessler, author of *The End of Overeating*. He makes an excellent argument that salt, sugar and fat, when expertly combined (think Ice Cream Sundae) can lead to "conditioned hyper-eating."

I believe many "How Much" eaters are truly addicted to the salt, sugar and fats in our food, and while they don't have an eating disorder (according to Dr. Kessler), they find it very hard to stop overeating. Don't confuse these conditioned hyper-eaters with "Why" eaters. Their emotions may not come into play at all since it's purely a physiological response to the food ingredients. The key for these people is to stop eating foods loaded with salt, sugar and fat and to restructure their food cravings towards the plant based foods they were designed to eat. See the Food Stoplight Charts in Chapter 20.

It is important to note that modern science has been very successful in developing birth control products so that we can enjoy sex without procreation. Although researchers are continually trying to devise methods for us to enjoy food without gaining weight, they aren't even close to achieving the same success. We do have various surgical procedures available such as stomach banding and intestinal diversion, but they only come with serious risk, significant pain, limited success and great expense. As of this writing, there truly is no easy fix or any realistic way to outsource our weight loss.

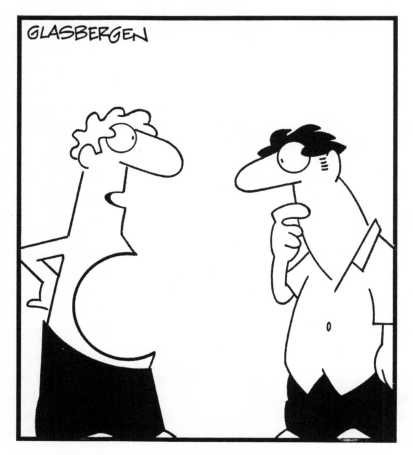

GLASBERGEN

"Belly button enlargement is a popular alternative to other types of weight loss surgery."

"Why" and "How Much" eaters share many of the same characteristics. Many people tell me they have a hard time determining which one they are. I explain that "Why" eaters eat too much food because they eat for the wrong reasons, generally in response to emotional issues throughout the day. "How Much" eaters may be fairly consistent in consuming just three meals a day, but the amounts or portion sizes are so big they are getting too many calories.

I've met numerous "How Much" eaters that eat a reasonably healthy diet, yet are still overweight. It really is quite easy to consume more calories than you burn, even if you only eat healthy, low calorie food. I see many of these people in my local gym. They are getting every bit as good a workout as I am, but they are still overweight. It's only when they address **how** they get those extra calories that they will begin to lose weight.

While most of us have a predominate factor responsible for our overweight condition, it's possible to have a combination of two or more factors. Many "How Much" eaters also need to address "What" foods they are eating. Your self-assessment can help you discover if this is the case for you.

The bottom line, of course, is that all overweight individuals ultimately consume too many calories. It's the reasons that we eat all those extra calories that are different for each of us. While we must learn to consume fewer calories to lose weight, how we achieve it can be different for each person.

> While we must learn to consume fewer calories to lose weight, how we achieve it can be different for each person.

"How Much" eaters really need to focus on portion size. I don't advocate counting calories or points as *Weight Watchers* does because it's not realistic to do it for the rest of your life. I would be remiss if I didn't mention *Weight Watchers* since I've met so many of their devotees at my seminars and in my social circles. *Weight Watchers* doesn't require you to buy their food (and most people don't), but the food you do eat has to be converted into a running daily / weekly tally of points. Is this something you want to do for the rest of your life?

I do acknowledge that among commercial weight loss programs, *Weight Watchers* does seem to have the most loyal following. Because of this, I've studied *Weight Watchers* participants very closely, and have noted their near universal desire to lose more weight.

A 2009 *CBS MoneyWatch* review reported that *Weight Watchers* was the best out of the eight they studied, was the oldest national weight loss program, and least expensive ($6 to $10 per pound lost). Remembering that this is the best out of the most popular weight loss programs, the *MoneyWatch* report also indicated that participants "lost an average of about five percent of their body weight (10 pounds)"….and that "two years later, they had kept about <u>half</u> the weight off." Is this what you're shooting for?

> When you come right down to it, only you can solve your own weight problem.

I'm also not crazy about paying 10-15 bucks to get weighed. Yes, they provide a great support system, but when you come right down to it, only you can solve your own weight problem. If this support system, or any of the commercial weight loss world's offerings work for you in delivering <u>permanent</u> weight loss, I'd say go for it. Just realize that ultimate success, no matter what program you use, depends solely on <u>you</u>.

One of the things I learned early during my journey was that all of the commercial weight loss programs are in the same business: making money! Therefore they are designed to generate constant cash flow. They make money even if you never lose a pound. The same *MoneyWatch* report quoted above indicated the following costs, per plan, to lose 20 pounds:

eDiets – $1,556 for 13 weeks

Jenny Craig – $1,070 to $2,120 depending on how fast you lose weight

Nutrisystem – About $706 for 8 weeks of food on the standard plan

Medifast – $480 plus the cost of your own groceries for the "lean and mean" meals

In the Zone Delivery – $4,480 for 16 weeks of food

My goal was to write a book that works for everyone. Yes, my method may be harder than outsourcing your problem to *Jenny Craig*, but it will work. You'll achieve permanent results and you'll never spend another dime on weight loss.

If you use the method of self-assessment and adhere to the Five Basic Truths, you'll find that through experimentation, trial and error and a little practice, you'll know how much and what kinds of food you can eat. If you're losing weight, you've got it right, and when you do reach your target weight, you'll use the same skills to eat the same number of calories that you burn daily. When you effortlessly match the calories you're eating to the calories you're burning, you'll find you can maintain your target weight forever. Yes it's harder to do this at first, but it's the only way that will allow you to achieve permanent weight loss.

> The beauty of learning the principles in this book is that you can function in the real world.

When you master the process of matching calories eaten to calories burned, you'll find that this skill will serve you everywhere you go. I occasionally find myself in a situation where the food choices are limited. When I was invited to a beach party where there was only beer and bratwurst, I enjoyed both. But knowing that this would provide more fat and calories than I would normally consume, I made adjustments in my food choices for the rest of the weekend. The beauty of learning the principles in this book is that you can function in the real world. Yes, I do exercise self-discipline, but I have not sentenced myself to a life devoid of fun food.

The experimentation and trial and error process I advocate, while simple in concept, usually generates the most questions at my seminars. Months later when I meet attendees who've lost weight, they claim it was the easiest thing they've ever done. The key is to stick with it long enough to "figure it out" as I did. Most people don't remember the initial stages, only how easy it seemed when they got it right!

I've met people who tell me they have been doing all the "right things" yet they haven't lost any weight. In the kindest way possible, I tell them that if they were doing the right things, they'd be losing weight. The problem is that only they can figure out the right things. If you're not honest with yourself, how are you going to do this? Only **you** can figure out what combination of skills or principles, all discussed in this book, will work for your weight loss. Your Guiding Star in Chapter 27 will help you keep track of what works for you.

> That's why trial and error is so important; every person is different and needs different solutions.

On the *Biggest Loser* TV show, you observe how tough Jillian is with the participants. She has to be because so many people are unwilling to put forth the initial effort required to understand weight loss. Losing weight is not hard! What is hard is figuring out how to lose weight. That's why trial and error is so important; every person is different and needs different solutions.

The *Biggest Loser* participants start out in a very controlled environment where they learn how to lose weight, but the real results only happen after they go home and prove that they can succeed in the real world. Many of us have seen the unbelievable results these men and women achieve, proving that any of us can achieve permanent weight loss if we put forth the initial effort to understand how weight loss works. Unfortunately, we don't have Jillian to help us.

Even though I correctly identified myself as a "What" eater, figuring out which foods I could still eat and enjoy while simultaneously losing weight took some time and effort. Once I determined a workable combination of foods, beverages, sleep and exercise that didn't violate the Five Basic Truths, it was like I was on autopilot. I was still monitoring the gauges, but the actual losing weight part was relatively easy.

Listening to many people discuss their weight issues, I've learned that many of us aren't willing to make the initial investment of time and effort to figure it out. The commercial weight loss programs take us right to the losing weight part, because they know we don't have the patience to figure it out for ourselves. If we could just understand what a huge payoff this effort produces, we all would be committed to working our way through the trial and error process. There's no other way to succeed in weight loss. If you're not willing to put forth the effort, you'll never achieve permanent weight loss.

If you're having difficulty figuring it out, it can help to change your focus or ultimate goal. For many of us, approaching a problem from a different or new perspective can really help. Many people achieve weight loss success when they change their focus from trying to lose weight to trying to live healthier. When they do this, weight loss becomes just one of the many by-products (more energy, less stress, etc) of a healthier lifestyle. When I think about it, my sister's death motivated me not only to lose weight, but also to pursue a healthier lifestyle.

> There's no other way to succeed in weight loss. If you're not willing to put forth the effort, you'll never achieve permanent weight loss.

Your Focus Areas as a "How Much" Eater:

1. Learn the three "Ps" - Portion size, Planning and Practice.

   • Be honest with yourself about the amount of food you eat and cut your portions by at least a third.

   • Plan your meals and decide ahead of time what you'll eat, especially when you will be away from home.

   • Practice eating the right foods. Avoid foods loaded with salt, sugar and fat. As you steer yourself away from eating the wrong foods, you'll find you're not craving food all the time.

2. Eat more slowly. Many "How Much" eaters really eat much too fast.

3. Choose low calorie-dense foods. This will allow you to eat the same amount (volume) of food that you are used to eating and still lose weight.

4. Exercise, but don't assume that just because you're hitting the gym, you can eat as much as you want.

5. Choose drinks carefully. Note the calories in those beverages!

An interesting point: If you watch the *Biggest Loser* on television, see if you can identify the "What," "Why," and "How Much" eaters. You may find it easier than you think!

8

"How Much You Move" Eaters

The **"How Much You Move"** folks make up a bigger and bigger portion of today's overweight population (pun intended!). We simply don't get enough exercise in our current environments in relation to the calories we consume. Many of us work in a sedentary environment where there are few chances for any measurable exercise.

The modern conveniences of elevators, along with fast food restaurants and cafeterias that serve high calorie-dense foods also contribute to the challenge of maintaining an appropriate weight for our height. Our busy and stressful modern lives can also cause us to seek the comfort and ease that comes in a widely available variety of fast or pre-packaged foods and beverages. If we don't get enough exercise, we can easily exceed the calories in (eaten) over the calories out (burned). Your self-assessment log should reveal how much exercise, if any, you are getting.

In my seminars I tell people to vehemently protect their ability to move. If you have an injury or condition that prevents you from participating, pain-free, in at least daily brisk walking, weight loss can be very challenging.

It's not just the sedentary workforce in this country that is overweight, however. Many folks who have jobs that entail almost constant movement are also overweight, showing that exercise alone is not the key to losing weight. Exercise is important for everyone, but it's not the only weight loss tool for everyone.

Remember, exercise wasn't even a factor in my ability to lose weight as I was already engaged in an aggressive workout routine, yet I still gained weight year after year. Of course, if I hadn't been exercising I would have weighed a lot more. There's an entire chapter on exercise and I encourage you to read it. If you're not currently engaged in an exercise regimen, check with your doctor first, then get started.

The bottom line is that we all must exercise for good health, longevity, quality of life and the prevention of heart disease and strokes.

The bottom line is that we all must exercise for good health, longevity, quality of life and the prevention of heart disease and strokes. Many of us probably need a little more exercise and better nutrition no matter where the self-assessment process points us to focus our weight loss efforts. We have to exercise, especially if we want to eat the fun calories. The human body requires movement. Exercise, in some form, is the key.

Your Focus Areas as a "How Much You Move" Eater:

1. Exercise is critical if you have discovered you don't have enough activity in your daily routine. See the chapter on exercise (Chapter 13) for a full explanation.

2. Most people who find they are predominately a "How Much You Move" type person actually have fairly good diets. If you didn't, you would've discovered that you're predominately a "What, Why, or How Much" eater.

3. Don't give up sleep to start an exercise regimen. That's counterproductive.

4. Exercise alone won't make up for too many extra calories. Eating fewer calorie-dense foods can really accelerate the weight loss process.

5. Don't use sports drinks just because you're exercising. They have tons of carbohydrates, calories and sodium. Plain water is best unless you're competing in extreme physical challenges such as the *Ironman Triathlon*.

As I said in the Foreword, a weight loss journey is principally a cerebral exercise. Clearly, there is a lot to know about how the body works, what foods and drinks are the best and the best ways to exercise. They're all covered in the following chapters. Quite frankly, it's really not that complicated, but there is a lot to learn. Once you understand the Five Basic Truths and conduct your personal self-assessment, implement the practices in the following chapters and see which ones produce the best results.

Your Guiding Star in Chapter 27 will be a useful tool to record what works the best. My contention is that if you can discover the top five skills for you (reward is the fifth on my five-pointed star), you'll be well on your way to permanent weight loss. We're all different, so while the skills are all valid weight loss tools, some will work for you better than others. Only you can figure out the best ones for you and then apply them.

Finally, I've found that most people don't really believe that they can lose weight. In my seminars, I explain that it was only after I had lost more than 23 pounds that I finally was convinced that I could be successful. Don't let this happen to you. You were designed to be slender. Once you implement the practices in this book (yes, it'll require a little effort), your body will return to its appropriate weight. I promise!

I can't emphasize enough the importance of conducting your own personal self-assessment and being truly mentally prepared before you begin the weight loss process.

9

I'm Overweight – So What?

I have met people who tell me they are "happy" or "comfortable" with their weight and that the world will have to accept them the way they are. While I'll always accept someone for who they are, and understand we are all wonderfully different, I now know that being overweight is a serious threat to their health. I also realize none of us were designed to be overweight.

> I also realize none of us were designed to be overweight.

Our early ancestors didn't even understand the concept of being overweight. They spent so much time and energy trying to stay warm and fed that it was impossible for them to store more than a few pounds of body fat. This is the legacy we have inherited as human beings.

Our Paleolithic ancestors burned one calorie for every nine calories of food they hunted or gathered. Early farmers expended one calorie for every 53 calories of crops they raised, and today we burn one calorie for every 210 calories worth of food we buy while grocery shopping. And you think you have a hard life?

Although it's now possible, even easy, to store excess fat, the human body is not well adapted to this condition. The result is that we've seen a rise in an incredible array of diseases that are directly attributable to being overweight.

Study after study has shown that being overweight (BMI over 25), or obese (BMI 30 and above), significantly increases your incidence of heart disease, diabetes, strokes and cancers of the breast, colon, prostate, uterus, esophagus and kidneys. The increase is 50 percent in some cases! These are all serious diseases that will significantly affect your longevity and your quality of life. See the Body Mass Index (BMI) chart on page 170 to determine your BMI. You may be quite surprised.

Don't confuse accepting being overweight with being happy. You can't be fat and happy. Although I dislike that term, you'll hear many people claim they are, in fact, "fat and happy." I contend that it's impossible for any human to be so. If you've met me, you'll see I'm bald. Now given the choice, I'd choose having hair rather than being bald. I'm not happy about it, but I've accepted it. Other than having an extensive hat collection and spending a fortune on sunscreen, being bald won't affect my longevity or quality of life. On the other hand, being overweight would. We should never confuse the wonderfully different bodily attributes (baldness, red hair, blue eyes, tall, short, etc.) with being overweight. Being overweight isn't a natural condition for us humans!

I have often told people that I wouldn't accept anything to go back to my old weight. You could offer me 50 million dollars and I wouldn't do it. I was 34 pounds overweight and I now feel like I've been liberated from prison. I saw the pain and anguish in my sister's eyes, the result of her overweight condition.

> Being overweight isn't a natural condition for us humans!

Tell yourself right now, "Achieving an appropriate weight for my height is the most important mission in my life." For so many of us, realizing the importance of losing weight is a critical first step in committing to do something about it. When we can tie a reason for losing weight to an ultimate result, the effects are powerful. I've heard reasons for wanting to lose weight range from being able to ride a roller coaster with friends to gaining confidence to start dating.

Finally, as I said earlier, no one mentions what our acceptance of being overweight is doing to our children. If you're overweight, chances are good that your kids will be too. Remember what it was like back in elementary and high school? It's hard enough without having to be subjected to the ridicule of being overweight.

Even if the other kids don't tease your children, the loss of self-esteem, confidence and the potential to develop unhealthy eating habits can plague them throughout their adult lives. Not only will they be afflicted with life-threatening diseases earlier in life, but they'll also be subjected to social disadvantages and possible discrimination in the job market. The worst possible ramifications include eating disorders, such as anorexia nervosa and bulimia, and the potential for depression and suicide.

You'll never realize how closely your children watch your actions, as opposed to listening to your words, then when they see you taking health and nutrition seriously. I saw how much influence my weight loss journey had on my two boys. Today, my oldest hardly eats the school lunch and prefers to eat the fruit, nuts and yogurt he takes from home. My youngest proudly announced that the first ingredient in the dry cereal he selected is whole grain oats. They have watched me very closely and have seen the incredible transformation I've made. I'm certain that they will carry the skills they've learned into a healthy adulthood.

10
Losing Weight – The Basics

After I was mentally prepared and realized where to focus my weight loss efforts, I determined that I needed to better define "weight loss." As a graduate of the Naval War College, I knew how to deconstruct large, complex problems into (pardon the pun) small digestible parts.

I discovered that losing weight is defined as changing the body's ratio of muscle mass to stored fat. I once read that the quickest way to lose 10 pounds was to cut off your head, but that clearly would be counterproductive in a weight loss journey. I needed to lose stored fat while maintaining or increasing my muscle mass*. I needed to discover why the body stored fat in the first place, because I knew that after I drank sufficient water so that my body was properly hydrated, my body got rid of the excess. Why wasn't the same true for fat?

> I discovered that losing weight is defined as changing the body's ratio of muscle mass to stored fat.

What I discovered was fascinating. The body is an amazing machine magnificently adapted to our ancestors environment. In spite of our many attempts to control it and force it to lose weight, the body has developed a survival mechanism that has served it well for millions of years. In short, the body stores fat to survive.

Early man and woman gained one-two pounds each spring and summer to prepare for winter. When the weather got cold

---

*Most commercial weight loss plans incorrectly focus on just losing / burning fat. Unfortunately, after yo-yo dieting (losing and regaining weight), many people discover that they have lost so much muscle mass, and eventually gained so much weight, that they find it difficult to re-establish an exercise program. Losing weight requires that we focus on both losing fat and building (or at least maintaining) muscle mass.

and the food supply shrank, this stored fat kept them alive. This "storing of fat" response was developed over many thousands, probably millions, of years. While we don't need to store as much fat anymore, our bodies have not adapted to our near-constantly available food supply. It will take literally tens of thousands of years to adapt, far too long to help us with our own weight loss!

One of the exercises I conduct during my speaking engagements is to ask people to remember what they weighed at their optimum weight. "What did you weigh when you graduated from high school or when you got married? Subtract that weight from your current weight. Now divide the difference by the number of years it's been." Often the result is between one and two pounds per year.

Another way to calculate out how much you've gained per year...

1. _____ Your weight now

− _____ Subtract your weight in high school/ when you got married

= _____ Difference in pounds

2. Difference in pounds _____ divided by _____ years since high school / got married = _____ number of pounds gained per year.

In my case, I was in my best physical condition when I graduated from Aviation Officer Candidate School in 1981. I was 5'11" and weighed 169 pounds the day I was commissioned an officer in the Navy. In 2002 I weighed 203 pounds. I had gained 34 pounds in 21 years, or just a little more than one and a half pounds per year.

A lot of us have gained one to two pounds per year. It creeps up on us without our being aware it's there. If you have, it's an important clue into why you're overweight and what you'll need to do to lose it. People that have gained these one-two pounds per year are generally "What" and "How Much You Move" types. My "lose 30 pounds in 30 weeks regimen" will probably work well for you even if you need to lose 50 pounds or more.

I recently heard about a study that identified the three most effective diets. I won't name them here because they all had abysmal, generally less than five percent success rates. You wouldn't buy a $3,000 LED television if the salesperson told you there was only a one in 20 chance that the picture would look as good once you got it home. Yet we spend billions every year on diets that simply don't work for the majority of folks that buy them.

The study concluded that even with their poor success rates, all three diets had a common theme. They all recommended that you choose a diet that has you consume fewer calories than you burn each day. That is the only way to lose weight unless you go for the "chop off your head" approach.

As I stated in the previous chapter, how we go about consuming fewer calories each day is different for all of us. **To lose weight you must figure out how to continue to enjoy eating while simultaneously consuming fewer calories than you burn.** The good news is that once you are at an appropriate weight for your height, the calories you eat each day can equal the calories you burn.

It's this delicate balance of consuming fewer calories than you burn that causes dieters to fail. As I stated earlier, the body is smart. It's not going to let you starve yourself. If you've ever tried a starvation diet you know what I mean. I tried it and my body told me, "If you're not going to feed me, I'm not going to work."

Your body will slow down tremendously after missing just a few meals, or when the calorie count goes down suddenly. The body adjusts the calories burned very quickly to equal the calories consumed, and not surprisingly, the dieter is both miserable and doesn't lose any weight. This goes on for a few days, at best, and many dieters decide that they'll never lose any weight and give up. Sound familiar?

In order to lose weight you need to have an approximately 500 calorie deficit per day. That's right, eat 500 fewer calories a day than you burn, or burn 500 calories more a day than you eat. The body will respond to this slow decline in calories by tapping into your stored fat to make up the difference. Finding this balance can take a little trial and error, but becomes easier when you re-learn Basic Truth #3 and listen to the signals that your body is sending you.

I'll never advocate counting calories or points because that is something I'm just not willing to do for the rest of my life. Do you want to count points for the rest of your life? Remember Basic Truth #2? "Only make a lifestyle or diet change that you can do forever."

With this 500-calorie deficit approach, you generally can give up only a small portion of the food you're eating now. In fact, you can even eat more and still consume fewer calories if you eat the right foods (see the chapter on Calorie Density and the Food Stoplight Charts). If you're not currently exercising, you can give up 250 calories in food and add a 250 calorie workout to get the 500 calorie deficit. With this deficit, most people who've been consuming 2,000 calories a day can give up just 12.5 percent of their normal calories and still lose weight. That sounds doable, doesn't it?

The really good news is that moderate exercise, like brisk walking seems to work best for burning fat. The best time to exercise is at least 3-4 hours after you've eaten. With fewer carbs in your body, this moderate exercise seems to replicate that long-lost winter and the body switches to using stored fat. This is why exercising first thing in the morning (okay, have that cup of black coffee before you exercise) works best for so many people. I eat a healthy breakfast, work out at lunchtime and eat lunch at my desk afterwards.

Based on your schedule, you could work out before going home from work to have dinner. There are lots of possibilities, but you must <u>plan</u> for your daily exercise if you work in an office or sedentary setting. It may be helpful to schedule exercise times, like you would an appointment or meeting, in your *Day-Timer*, online calendar, or mobile device.

Initially during my weight loss journey, I found it worked best to eat four to five small meals per day, so I didn't quite reach that three-four hour point unless I worked out first thing in the morning. That's okay. The calories in = the calories out equation stills holds true. The stored fat in your body is used for fuel when you have no carbohydrates to burn. Your goal during a weight loss journey is to burn fat, so it makes sense to develop a workout routine that optimizes this fat-burning process.

Today, I only eat three times a day and often go four-five hours before I start my workout. As I refined my diet and steered away from processed and high glycemic index foods, I was better able to manage my blood sugar and didn't get hungry as fast or need to eat as often. This was really key for me in maintaining my weight loss. See Chapter 21 on the Glycemic Index for a full explanation.

No matter how you do it, a 500 calorie deficit per day equals 3,500 calories per week, which is exactly what you need to burn to lose one pound of fat. It's amazing how that works. You can work the math and quickly see that anything more than about one to two pounds per week is too difficult unless you're accepted onto the next *Biggest Loser* show. The participants on that show work out six-eight hours a day, have lots of fat to burn, and eat nearly perfect diets. Any other claims, like burning fat while you sleep if you take a certain pill, or losing 10 pounds in a week while still eating French fries is just plain baloney.

Unfortunately, the opposite is very possible. You really can gain weight faster than you can take it off. If you normally burn 2,000 calories a day, you can cut down to 1200-1400 calories (not recommended), although it may be very difficult. However, if you go on a vacation cruise, you can very easily consume 6,000 calories a day or more, especially if you indulge is very high calorie-dense foods. If you spend just a single week consuming 6,000 calories per day, you'll be eight pounds heavier when you come home (extra 4,000 x 7 = 28,000 ÷ 3,500 = 8 lbs.). Those eight pounds will take two months to burn off. Some vacation, huh?

> You really can gain weight faster than you can take it off.

No matter what reason you're out of balance (What, Why, How Much or How Much You Move), the only way to lose weight is to burn fat. If you're currently engaged in a regular workout routine and are still overweight, it's because you're consuming too many calories. That's why I designed the self-assessment to determine if it is "What" you're eating, "Why" you are eating, or "How Much." Only you can figure this out. This is where many of the commercial weight loss programs come up short. The fact remains though; the way to lose weight is the same for everyone. Burn more calories than you consume. There's no getting around that. How we individually approach this is what is different!

> The fact remains though; the way to lose weight is the same for everyone. Burn more calories than you consume.

A 500 calorie deficit per day will burn one pound of fat per week only if it's a deficit from your normal calorie output. If your burn 2,000 calories a day, and regularly eat and drink 3,000 calories a day, you need to cut back 500 calories below what you burn. That means down to 1,500 calories per day, or the calorie burn via exercise has to go up. This is doable for most people, but you'll need to combine good nutrition with low calorie density foods, the right drink choices, exercise and sufficient sleep.

One final thought: I've noticed how personality profiles affect individuals' ability to lose weight. Many of us know our *Myers-Briggs Type Indicator (MBTI)*. I'm an ESTJ and my wife is an ENFP. Though we're both **E**xtroverts, I'm more of a **S**ensing, **T**hinking, and **J**udging type person. She's i**N**tuitive, **F**eeling and **P**erceiving. I've found very little about this in my research, but can tell you that my wife and I view the world, and weight loss, very differently.

As an ESTJ, I'm pragmatic and when I see a *Snapple Ice Tea* I think of how good it will taste until I read how many calories are in a bottle. As an ENFP, my wife views it as how good the drink, or food, will make her feel. If one of the kids at her school gives her a cupcake, she feels compelled to eat it because she doesn't want to hurt the child's feelings. When the Girl Scouts show up at my front door selling cookies, I have to work really hard not to engage them in a lesson on the perils of refined grains and saturated fats. My wife will buy a box of every kind of cookie they're selling. This may be an area you need to examine, because how we handle these kinds of situations will affect our success in a weight loss journey.

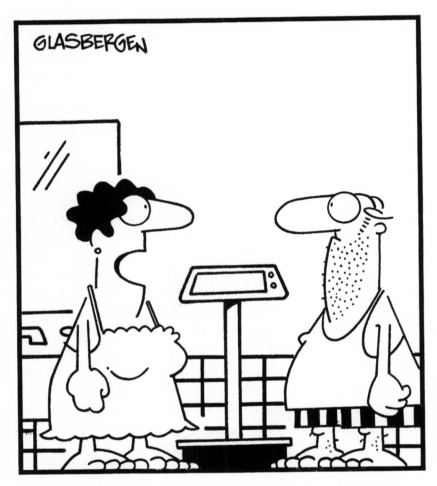

"Why does it take 6 weeks to lose 5 pounds,
but only 1 day to gain it all back?"

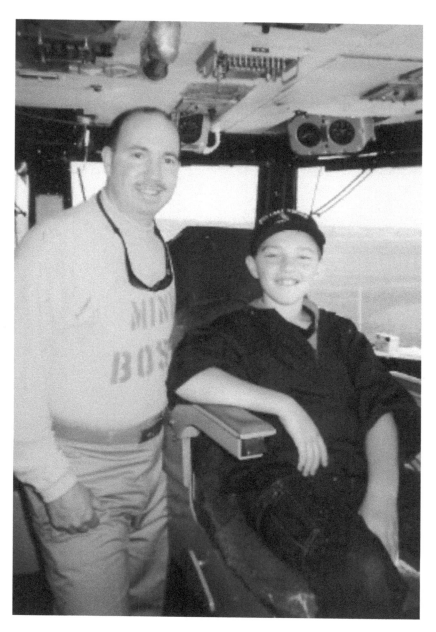

I'm in the tower of the USS CARL VINSON in 2001 with my then 10-year old son, Edmond, when I weighed more than 200 pounds.

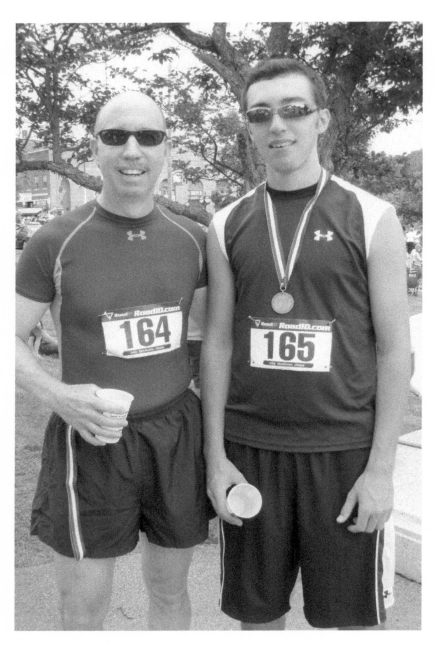

This was in July, 2007 when I was back to my 1981 weight of 169 lbs. That's my son, Ed at age 16, 6' 2" tall, and 170 lbs.

11
It's Five O'Clock Somewhere

Jimmy Buffet perfectly immortalized the wonderfully relaxing feeling of having an icy cold beverage on a warm, balmy day. *Margarittaville* was his destination of choice, and it didn't matter what time of day he arrived. If you've ever had a frozen margarita, mid-day, during a vacation to the islands, you've been to *Margaritaville*.

With my apologies to Jimmy Buffet, it's time for a dose of reality on how our drink choices affect our ability to lose weight. There are two key things I learned concerning the drink choices I made during my weight loss journey. First, early man had only one drink choice, water. Second, we were designed to get calories only from food. Consequently, our bodies adapted to water, and it's still the best fluid to drink. Throughout time, we've developed a few more choices: milk from animals, juice from fruit, and relatively recently in the grand scheme of things, soft drinks, coffee, tea, beer and my favorite, wine.

I found a web-site (www.thefatmanwalking.com) through my research that chronicled Steve Vaught's weight loss journey. His story was interesting, but the thing I remember most was that he called water "The fluid of change." He couldn't have spoken truer words.

Man has been on earth for millions of years according to the *History Channel*. Again, for the majority of those years, water was the only available beverage. Beer and wine have existed fewer than 10,000 years. *Coke* and other soft drinks have only been available for a little more than 100 years. Even at that, when I was a kid, a *Coke* was a treat, not a daily staple, and only came in a six-ounce bottle.

The American Journal of Preventive Medicine published a study in 2004 that showed how much our drinking habits have changed. We drink twice the fruit drinks and alcohol than we did in the 1970s. Soda consumption has nearly tripled at a time when we're drinking 40 percent less milk. *Starbucks* aficionados might be interested to learn that coffee consumption, a relatively healthy drink choice, has increased a mere nine percent in spite of its wide popularity. Why is this important? Because many of today's drink choices are laden with tons of calories, even fruit juices and many so-called coffee drinks.

Another thing I learned was that we have developed separate hunger and thirst mechanisms. Barry M. Popkin, who heads the Division of Nutrition Epidemiology in the School of Public Health at the University of North Carolina, has done a great deal of work on this. He believes that we were designed so that food wouldn't quench thirst and fluids wouldn't satisfy hunger.

Fast-forward to today and it is possible to get a drink at *Starbucks* that has nearly 800 calories. Not recognizing this as food, our bodies will still want the same daily amount of food. Quite easily we can drink, rather than eat, nearly half a day's typical calories (about 2,000 calories a day for the average American).

> Remember, during a weight loss journey you still want to, and must, eat!

If we don't watch our drink choices, we can consume many more calories than we can burn each day. In fact, you can markedly reduce your calorie intake during a weight loss journey just by making better drink choices. While at work, I switched from soft drinks, *Gatorade* and fruit drinks, to plain water and truly believe that this simple change had a profound effect on my results. Remember, during a weight loss journey you still want to, and must, eat! Developing a 500 calorie deficit can really be aided by carefully selecting the fluids you drink, **thereby saving the calories for food**.

Now I can hear you saying, "I'll just drink zero-calorie diet sodas." Not so fast. Remember, your body is smarter than you are. It's expecting water with zero calories, not chemicals with zero calories. If you drink regular soda, switching to diet drinks <u>can</u> help you lose weight since you'll be cutting out a significant number of empty calories. I switched to diet drinks from regular soda and then eventually changed to water as I felt better (listening to my body) and realized that water was better for me.

A 2008 study showed a link between diet sodas and metabolic syndrome*. The study couldn't identify the specific link, but one researcher suggested that people who are already overweight and eat unhealthy foods try to compensate by drinking diet sodas. The link could be as simple as that. Additionally, the jury is still out on the efficacy of the artificial sweeteners and the long term deleterious effects of drinking sodas. Keep in mind that many dark-colored colas contain chemicals and acids that are just not doing your body and stomach any good.

If there really were any evidence that diet sodas helped people lose weight we would see it splashed all over diet drink advertising. Yet we hear very little on the subject from the diet drink industry. Recent studies are now pointing to the possibility that the artificial sweeteners in diet drinks actually stimulate hunger, the exact opposite of what you are trying to achieve. My advice is to give up the diet sodas and switch to water!

<u>**Meal replacement shakes**</u> fall somewhere in the middle, like soup, between solid food and fluids. Barry Popkin reports that soup, even broth, is probably registered as food by the body. Why or how, we just don't know. Meal replacement shakes probably fit in here somewhere, but I don't recommend them (see my recommendations on the next page).

* Metabolic Syndrome is a group of (metabolic) risk factors all present in a single individual. The risk factors include abdominal obesity, high blood pressure, insulin resistance (or glucose intolerance), and blood abnormalities that include high triglycerides, high LDLs (Low Density Lipoproteins) and C-reactive protein, and low HDLs (High Density Lipoproteins). This is a serious life threatening condition that needs to be immediately addressed. The best thing you can do is to lose weight if your doctor has told you that you have Metabolic Syndrome.

A weight loss journey is primarily a journey of discovery. Eating meals sent to your door or drinking a shake to replace a meal is not helping you learn critical food choice skills. Eating should be in response to true hunger and include <u>conscious</u> food choices. You have to actually think about your nutrition and what's best for you in a world where there are so many choices. By educating myself on what was good, and what was not so good for my health and nutrition, I was able to start making the right choices.

<u>**Sports drinks**</u> (*Gatorade*, etc.) are useful if you're running a marathon. They're designed to replace vital bodily fluids when loss occurs during heavy exertion and perspiration. But if you're just hitting the gym for a daily workout, water is still the best choice.

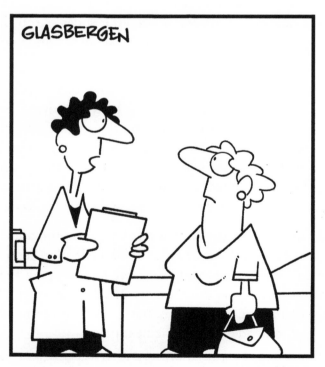

"The only diet shake I recommend is the shake your booty makes when you exercise!"

My recommendations for daily drink choices:

Water - (0 calories). The average person needs the equivalent of about four 16-ounce / half liter bottles of water per day. The water in your coffee and other drinks, plus the fruits and vegetables you eat, count as part of this amount. The old "Eight, 8-ounce glasses of water per day" rule always seems to leave out this important fact. If you're listening to your body (e.g. notice signs of dehydration, feeling thirsty, dark yellow colored urine, etc.) you'll know if you need more or less fluid.

Coffee / Tea - (8 oz. = 0 - 50 calories). Black coffee has about five calories, but cream and sugar raise the calories up to 50 per cup, depending upon how much you use.

Milk - (8 oz. fat free = 80 calories; 1 percent milk = 100 calories). Fat-free dairy foods (yogurt, cottage cheese, etc) are great substitutes for milk and will provide even more needed calcium while counting as food calories.

100% Fruit Juices - (8 oz. = 40 - 160 calories). The calories can really start to add up here, but orange / grapefruit juice (110 calories) are vitamin and anti-oxidant rich and very beneficial. So is pomegranate juice (160 calories) and cranberry juice (140 calories for the cranberry juice cocktail / 40 for the light version). I cut the pomegranate and cranberry juice in half with water as they are too sweet for me straight out of the bottle. This saves half the calories and I don't go broke buying pomegranate juice.

Alcohol – Beer (12 oz. = approx. 160 calories), Wine (5 oz = 130 calories). The much-loved frozen Margarita (6 oz = 250 calories). See the next chapter on Alcohol for a full discussion of consuming alcohol during a weight loss journey.

Your goal during a weight loss journey should be to consume no more than 10-15 percent of your calories from fluids.

Your goal during a weight loss journey should be to consume no more than 10-15 percent of your calories from fluids. That means that if you are aiming for 1500 calories a day for a 500 calorie deficit, you can have between 150 and 225 calories from beverages. Some people profess that drinking only water is best during a weight loss journey. Basic Truth #2 says never make a change you can't / won't do forever, so I view this as counter-productive. You won't just drink water for the rest of your life, so why do it just to lose weight?

What happens when you go back to your favorite drinks? Truth be known, I drank wine during my entire weight loss journey because I flatly refused to give it up. At 130 calories a glass, it wasn't hard to stick with my calorie limit even if I drank a little more than a glass. I stuck with the recommendations above and was fairly successful by drinking water, black coffee, and milk with my cereal in the morning and wine with dinner.

You can have any combination of drink choices providing you don't go much above your calorie limit. See my Calorie Guide to the Most Popular Drinks on this and the following pages.

Calorie Guide for the Most Popular Drinks
(listed from least to most calories)

Note: All drink sizes are eight ounces unless specified otherwise. Data were derived from various company websites, caloriesindrinks.com and thecaloriecounter.com.

Water or club soda.. 0
Polar Fruit flavored water 0
Diet soda 0
Starbucks Pike Place Roast (black) Coffee (16 oz)............. 5

Tea, with 2 sugar packs 20
Propel Water 25
Coffee, cream / 1 sugar 30
Ocean Spray light cranberry 40
Tropicana light orange juice 50
Minute Maid OJ (light) 50
Campbell's tomato juice 50
V8 Juice (11.5 oz.) 70
Milk, fat free 80
Yoplait light smoothie 90
O'Douls Amber (12 oz.) 90
Milk, 1% 100
Sierra Mist soda (8 oz. size) 100
Monster Energy (8 oz. single serving) 100
Coors Lite (12 oz.) 102
Full Throttle 110
Red Bull 110
Beer, light (12 oz.) 110
Orange juice (regular) 110
Hawaiian Punch 110
Starbuck's Cappuccino, with whole milk, tall (12 oz.) 110
Amp Energy 114
Hype Energy 114
SoBe Energy 120
Apple juice or 2% milk 120
Wine, white (5 oz.) 120
Glaceau Vitamin Water 125
Gatorade (20 oz.) 130
Starbucks Caffe' Latte, with skim milk (16 oz.) 130
Wine, red (5 oz.) 130
Cranberry juice cocktail 140
Silk Chocolate Soymilk 140
Single malt scotch (2 oz.) 140
Coke Classic (12 oz.) 140
Budweiser (12 oz.) 145

Sierra Nevada Bigfoot Beer (12 oz.) 320

Nestle' Nesquik Chocolate Milk (16 oz.)......................... 330

Tropicana Fruit Fury Twister (20 oz.)............................... 340

Arizona Rx Energy (23 oz.)... 345

Arizona Kiwi Strawberry (23 oz.) 345

Dunkin Donuts Coffee Coolatta, with cream (16 oz.) 350

Starbucks Mocha Frappuccino w/ whipped cream (16 oz.) 370

TCBY Fruithead Smoothie (20 oz.)................................... 410

7-Eleven Super Big Gulp, Coke (44 oz) 410

Auntie Anne's Wild Cherry Lemonade Mixer (32 oz.) 470

Starbucks Iced Double Chocolaty Chip
     with whipped cream (24 oz.) 520

Carnation Instant Breakfast (8.45 oz.) 560

McDonald's Chocolate Triple Shake (small 16 oz.)......... 580

Starbucks Iced Peppermint White Chocolate Mocha
     with whole milk & whipped cream (24 oz.) 720

Burger King vanilla shake (32 oz.).................................. 820

Dairy Queen Caramel MooLatte (24 oz.) 870

Red Lobster Lobsterita (24 oz.) 890

Baskin-Robins ice cream soda (28.6 oz.) 960

Baskin-Robbins vanilla shake (24 oz.) 980

Krispy Kreme Lemon Sherbet Chiller Frozen
     Fruit Drink (20 oz.) 980

McDonald's Chocolate Triple Thick Shake
     (large, 32 oz.) 1,160

Smoothie King Peanut Power Plus Grape Smoothie
(40 oz.) 1,498

Smoothie King Chocolate or Strawberry The Hulk
     (32 oz.)... 1,520

Cold Stone PB&C Milkshake.................................... 2,010

Which "Grande" Drink would you choose?

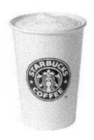 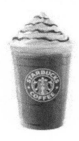 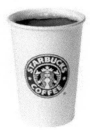

16oz Latte   Double Chocolate Chip   Black Coffee
                    Frappucino Blended Beverage

Choices count! All are the same "Grande" (medium)
16 oz. size, but the calories are vastly different.
Which did you chose?

Calories:
    Latte (nonfat milk) - 130 calories / 5g fat
    Double Chocolate Chip Frappucino Blended Crème -
        410 calories / 20g fat
    Black Coffee – 5 calories / 0g fat

12

Alcohol

Although I've already covered drink choices and how they affect a weight loss journey in the previous chapter, the consumption of alcohol in American society demands a discussion all its own. Now if you're thinking I'm going to lecture you on the ill effects of drinking alcohol and recommend you stay away from it altogether, you're wrong. Figuring out how to consume alcohol so that it contributes to your overall good health is the key. Unfortunately, developing the self-discipline to drink responsibly eludes many of us.

The most important fact to accept about alcohol consumption is that if you have ever been addicted to drugs, or any other substance (including alcohol obviously), turn to the next chapter. Drinking alcohol is not for you. If you are younger than 21 years old, you can turn to the next chapter as well. Young bodies with young minds that have a sense of immortality and indestructibility don't mix well with alcohol.

Clearly, there are obvious drawbacks to drinking alcohol. Alcohol can be very addicting and unlike drugs, it's legal, socially accepted, and darned easy to get. Statistics show that most of the alcohol we drink in this country is consumed by a relatively small percentage of the population. It's also responsible for many of the deaths on our highways and a whole host of medical and social problems.

That being said, <u>responsible</u> consumption of alcohol can be conducive to good health. Drinking moderate amounts of alcohol has been proven, in varied studies, to reduce your risk for cardiovascular disease (heart attack and stroke), lower the incidence of type-2 diabetes, reduce cancer risk and prevent the onset of Alzheimer's disease. It seems the key to healthy alcohol consumption is to have a little bit each day. The most widely accepted standard for drinking alcohol is one drink per day for women and two for men.

A drink is generally defined as a 12-ounce. beer, a five-ounce glass of wine or one and a half ounces of distilled spirits. (Note: A 750 ML bottle of wine contains approximately five, five-ounce glasses). You can't bank your daily quota and then consume all seven or 14 drinks on Friday night. That's a bad idea even if you have a designated driver because it wipes out any health benefit from drinking alcohol. The key takeaway here is that moderate consumption is essential to get the health benefits from drinking alcohol.

This is especially true for women. The widely accepted *Women's Health Study* found that as little as two drinks per day for women increased the risk of breast cancer by 30 percent. The study also found a strong connection between alcohol consumption and breast cancer for post-menopausal women on hormone replacement therapy. The *Hutchinson Study* found that women who consumed alcohol anytime in the past 20 years also had the same 30 percent increase in breast cancer risk. Some studies suggest that the simple act of taking a daily multi-vitamin that contains 400 micrograms of folic acid may help reduce some of the risk for women.

Some studies have found that while drinking alcohol lowers heart disease risk, the benefits are not realized until after menopause for women. All of these facts combine to indicate that a woman needs to make a conscientious choice on how much alcohol, if any, she consumes when weighed against the risks.

Men don't get a pass on the health risks of drinking alcohol even if they are allowed that second drink each day. Studies have shown that alcohol use increases the risk of cancers of the mouth, throat, esophagus, liver and colon.

Finally, the most important fact to consider during a weight loss journey is that it may not be the calories in the alcohol you're drinking, but the calories in the food you're eating while you're drinking. I have found that a few drinks with dinner can make it a great deal harder to say "no" to that 1,000 calorie dessert. Drinking alcohol needs to be approached cautiously anytime, but especially so when you're trying to lose weight.

> It may not be the calories in the alcohol you're drinking, but the calories in the food you're eating while you're drinking.

13

Exercise

There seems to be as much misinformation out there about exercise as there is about nutrition. Our early ancestors wouldn't have understood today's concept of exercise any more than they would have comprehended being overweight. For most of their existence on earth, the very act of survival guaranteed sufficient exercise. In fact, they probably husbanded their energy, realizing they had to maintain it to hunt / gather food, stay warm and ward off predators.

> Regular exercise is important for both men and women, at all ages.

Fast-forward to the early 21st century. Our existence in countries such as the United States has changed dramatically. In a very short amount of time, it's become possible to survive (but not truly thrive) without expending much physical energy. We are literally left with no choice but to artificially add a seemingly useless expenditure of energy to stay healthy. Wouldn't you like to hook up all those exercise machines in your local gym to generate the power requirements of your house? Think of what that would do for your utility bill!

Regular exercise is important for both men and women, at all ages. Recently, a 2010 conference of breast cancer researchers in Barcelona Spain found that breast cancer risk for women in western cultures could be cut by a third if they ate less and exercised more. The same conference reported that obese women may have a 60 percent higher risk for all forms of cancer.

Once we accept that exercise is vital for healthy human existence, we can start to make it a regular part of our lives. It doesn't have to be drudgery. Many people claim they get addicted to that so-called "runners high" and don't feel well or have as much energy unless they get some exercise every day.

Today, as a 52 year old, I realize the importance of movement, even if it's the simple act of keeping the house clean. Now I can hear some of you saying there is no way I'm going back to cleaning the bathroom. I understand. I still hate mowing the lawn, so now I have my son do it. The point is that exercise doesn't always mean going to the gym and beating the daylights out of those expensive exercise machines. You just need to figure out how you are going to include more movement into your daily routine. Everything from cleaning the house, taking the stairs at work, going for a walk, participating in sports, throwing the ball with your kids, golfing, swimming, gardening and so forth, counts.

Think back to the log I encouraged you to start in Chapter 3. I also recommended that you log how much exercise you get each day. For many of us, recording how much we move is a wake-up call to the fact that we hardly get any exercise in a normal day. You may need to change this to achieve an appropriate weight for your height. See the Exercise Startup Checklist and Log on page 171 to help you get started.

Exercise means different things to most of us and we can get it in various ways, such as physical labor, play, or working out. An effective exercise regimen combines cardio or aerobic movement for your heart, lungs and muscles, weight lifting for strength, and stretching for flexibility. Consider adding this triad of effective exercise if you discover that you need to move and exercise more.

Triad of Effective Exercise

1. **Cardio / Aerobic** (brisk walking, running, participating in sports, working out on exercise machines, etc.)

2. **Weight Lifting** (free weights, machines, any heavy lifting at work, etc.)

3. **Stretching** (with or without exercise balls and Pilates bands, etc.)

Cardio work is best for losing weight. If you are <u>not</u> currently exercising, this is the place to start. But I can't emphasize this point enough: <u>start slowly</u>. After we finally decide we've had enough of being overweight, the biggest mistake many of us make is to completely overexert ourselves when we start an exercise program. The next day we are so sore we can hardly get out of bed. If you don't normally exercise, your muscles have atrophied to the point that it takes very little exertion to overstress them.

I recommend walking around the block <u>once</u> if you haven't exercised in years. If that feels all right, try two times the next day. In a month's time you'll be power walking 30-45 minutes and will have a hard time remembering when you didn't, or couldn't, exercise at all. A word of caution: If you have any pre-existing medical condition, joint problems or take medication, please check with your doctors first. They'll be able to tell you what types of exercise are best for you.

The best fat burning cardio exercise is brisk walking. <u>Walking</u> for 30-60 minutes three to four hours after you've eaten will force your body to switch to stored fat for fuel. For a 52-year old like me, that means the optimum rate is to reach about 100-115 heart beats per minute. The machines in your local gym typically have heart rate monitors and charts that show you the optimum fat burning heart rate for your age. Or count your heart beats the old-fashioned way:

> Stop exercising and immediately place your middle fingers on your opposite wrist below your thumb to feel your pulse. Count the beats for ten seconds and multiply by six. That's your heart rate.

Don't make the mistake that I see many people making. They get on a cardio machine and go at break-neck speed, believing that it's the best way to lose weight. I see their heart rates go up to 160-170 beats per minute. That's not only dangerous for some of us, but it's also impossible to maintain for 30-60 minutes. It might seem hard to believe, but a steady fat-burning pace of 80-120 beats per minute (depending on your age) is best for losing weight.

Study after study has shown that cardio work significantly affects the number of mitochondria in your muscles cells. Why is this important? Mitochondria are the tiny engines in your muscles that, when tuned up with aerobic exercise, burn fat instead of carbohydrates. And burning fat is exactly what you want to do! There's only one catch. The benefit is short-lived, so you have to exercise regularly, about three-four times a week, throughout your life.

The good news is that the benefit kicks in at about 50 percent of your maximum capacity heart rate. Maximum capacity is defined as 220 minus your age. The 50 percent point starts at about 84 heartbeats a minute for a 52-year old like me (220 - 52 = 168; 50 percent of 168 = 84). That's a very comfortable walking pace. You'll find that it doesn't take much effort to get your heart rate to this point, regardless of your age. Studies have even shown a benefit for folks in their seventies and beyond. If you're not currently participating in aerobic exercise, get the clearance from your doctor to do so and see if you don't start to feel more energized and less fatigued. I promise you will!

Weight lifting is also important to healthy living. That does not mean power-lifting as if you're training for the next Mr. or Ms. Universe title. Start with a very low weight that you can comfortably and smoothly lift eight times. As your muscles get used to the weight, you can increase from the eight repetitions to 15. Then add a little more weight and start at eight reps again. You'll be amazed at how fast your muscles will respond.

> Weight lifting is also important to healthy living.

Being "out of shape" is not only a literal

term meaning that your body doesn't have the dimensions you'd like it to have. When you walk up a flight of stairs and need to catch your breath, it's because your muscles are not as adept at processing oxygen as they once were when you were "in shape." Muscles are metabolically very costly for the body to maintain. It takes lots of calories to keep those muscles strong. Your body, in spite of all those extra calories stored as fat, is quite stingy and will not spend the calories to maintain muscles unless you provide a payout for the calories invested.

By strengthening your muscles through weight lifting, you're telling your body you're willing to invest the calories needed to maintain them. These muscles become tiny individual furnaces, consuming large quantities of calories. The bigger muscles understandably have a bigger demand for fuel. That is why the machines you see in the gym are so popular because they exercise the muscles that demand the most calories.

Many people like to use the elliptical trainer because it exercises the broad muscles in the legs, arms and shoulders with little impact on the joints (as opposed to running). Another benefit is that muscles demand additional calories for several hours after your workout is complete. Stoking these calorie-burning furnaces will really help you achieve a 500 calorie deficit each day.

> Stretching is important so that you'll maintain flexibility, especially as you age.

Stretching is important so that you'll maintain flexibility, especially as you age. It also ensures that you'll keep your muscles limber enough to exercise. You can't, or won't want to exercise if you've pulled or strained a muscle. There's a difference between warming up and stretching. Warming up for a workout includes moving all your limbs and joints to get blood flowing to the muscles. The elliptical trainer is helpful for this as long as you use it on a low setting. Stretch after you exercise when the muscles are warm so they stretch easily and help increase your overall flexibility.

You may be self-conscience when it comes to beginning a workout program. One spin around the local gym and any of us can be intimidated by the guys with big muscles or those young gals with impossibly hard bodies. Repeat after me: "It's not about them. It's not about them. It's about my weight loss journey." The only person that you should compare yourself to is the old pre-exercise you.

Very early in my weight loss journey I realized that even though I was exercising, my lifestyle was a far cry from that of early man. Sure, I still worked out at lunch each day, but I used all the free time the conveniences this modern world afforded me to relax, watch the ball game on TV, or to socialize with my friends. While there's nothing wrong with enjoying our free time in these ways, they're usually the times when we eat the most calorie-dense foods.

I still enjoy relaxing with friends, but now realize how too much of a good thing can be a recipe for weight gain. In America today, our free time almost always includes fattening food. While this chapter focuses on exercise, it's vital to understand that we can't exercise long enough, or hard enough, to make up for overindulgence in social-setting calories.

That being said, the bottom line is that you must get some form of exercise. There is no way you'll ever be able to achieve and maintain an appropriate weight for your height, or truly thrive, unless your daily routine includes some form of exercise.

> The bottom line is that you must get some form of exercise.

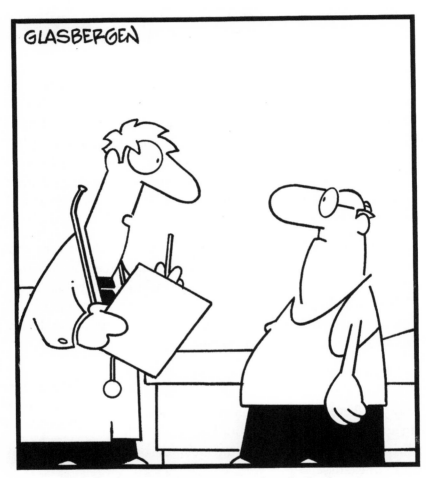

"What fits your busy schedule better,
exercising one hour a day or being
dead 24 hours a day?"

14

Sodium

The sodium, or salt, in our food is every bit as dangerous as the dense calories and fats we consume. In fact, the high level of sodium in our food is responsible for nearly 150,000 deaths in America each year. I only recently started to see an increase in press coverage about the high sodium levels in our food. If you travel to the United Kingdom (UK), you'll see many of the same foods you can purchase in America, but with much less sodium. Laws in the UK have been passed for reduced sodium, which are far overdue here in the U.S.

The FDA is finally "considering" their options to force food manufacturers to limit sodium in processed food. No sooner than this was announced, the Salt Institute's director for technical and regulatory affairs stated that regulation "would be a disaster for the public." Other lobbying groups even went as far as to say that the current understanding of how sodium affects our health is based on "junk science." This is what you are up against in a free society. It's up to you to find the truth.

Here's what my research turned up: Excess sodium in our food is responsible for raising our blood pressure which increases strokes and heart attacks. High blood pressure (above 120/80) is often referred to as the "silent killer." Since blood pressure screening is more prevalent these days, we tend to just treat it with medication. We don't address the root causes, which include the high amount of salt we ingest, our lack of exercise and our being overweight. I'm not saying blood pressure medication is bad for you. It's just that I see many people getting higher

> Excess sodium in our food is responsible for raising our blood pressure which increases strokes and heart attacks.

and higher doses of medication instead of addressing the amount of sodium in their diet, the fact that they're overweight, and that they get very little exercise.

I used to think that if I didn't use the salt shaker, I would really reduce the sodium in my diet. What I learned was that the sodium that came out of the salt shaker (zero for me these days) was a miniscule portion of the total sodium in my diet. Most of the salt in the average American diet comes from packaged food, prepared meals and restaurant fare. The USDA reports that 75 percent of the sodium Americans consume is added during food processing. Food manufacturers use lots of salt because it makes the food taste better and prolongs its shelf life.

The next time you go to the grocery store, check out the sodium content before you throw that box of prepared food, canned vegetables or soup into your grocery cart. You'll need to do a little math to avoid getting more sodium than you want. Many manufacturers will decide there are six servings in a box in order to report one sixth of the sodium, yet you'll prepare it for your family of four and get 50 percent more sodium in each serving.

> It's very easy to exceed the recommended maximum 2,400 mg of sodium per day if you eat packaged or prepared meals.

It's very easy to exceed the recommended maximum 2,400 mg of sodium per day if you eat packaged or prepared meals. In fact, the average American diet includes 3,500 mg of sodium per day. The USDA also reports that men consume nearly 1,300 mg more sodium per day than women. One stop at a fast food restaurant and you're probably half-way to your limit for the day.

If you have high blood pressure, diabetes, or are African American, you'll want to limit your daily sodium intake to 1,500 mg. This can be difficult with prepared, processed and fast foods, so you'll need to prepare the majority of your meals yourself. Be sure to include lots of fresh fruits and vegetables in your weekly meal planning (hey, we should be doing that anyway).

I tell people at my seminars that the best way to combat the high sodium content in our food is to "shop around the edges." Due to the realities of resupply logistics, all the fresh foods are located around the outside perimeter, or edges, of your local grocery store. Meats, dairy, fish and produce are found around the edges. You should only go into the aisles for soap and light bulbs. Now there are exceptions, of course, but not that many.

The high sodium products are in the aisles where you'll find canned goods (soup, vegetables), and packaged foods (rice mixtures, pasta dishes, salad dressings, lunch meats). Approach the frozen food aisle with caution as well. While there are some good choices there such as frozen low-sodium vegetables, there are also some of the things you may be tempted to buy like low-calorie TV dinners that contain an unbelievably high amount of sodium.

As I said, there are exceptions (*Cheerios*), but you'll need to read the labels to discover and buy the foods that do not pump you full of sodium. Sodium-filled products, like fats, are insidious. They're everywhere, and you need to be aware of food processing techniques, and in some cases, misleading product labels, to discover them.

Uncooked (fresh) chicken is a great example of unexpected sodium. Some manufacturers add both salt and water to keep the chicken moist, bringing a single serving (4 oz.) portion of unprepared chicken into the 400-700 mg of sodium range. This is before you season, marinate, salt or add a sauce to cook it!

Another way to mitigate the effect of sodium is to eat foods rich in potassium which can help lower your blood pressure without drugs, much the way I did. The good news is that high levels of potassium are found in some of the more popular and readily available foods. These include lean (low-salt) chicken, pork, baked white and sweet potatoes, as well as omega-3 rich foods like fish and Brussels sprouts.

Healthy fish choices include salmon, tuna, flounder and halibut. Potassium is also present in many easily transportable foods (think lunch in a *Ziploc* bag) like bananas, oranges, cantaloupe, grapes, raisins, watermelon, prunes and nuts (pistachios, almonds, peanuts).

I'm fairly adept at keeping my sodium intake low. I can tell because **my blood pressure has gone down each of the seven years I have been on my weight loss journey.** Without medication, my blood pressure is in the 110/70 range. Blood pressure at or below 120/80 is pretty good as long as it doesn't take ever increasing amounts of blood pressure medication to keep it there.

Have your blood pressure taken as often as you can and heed your doctor's advice on steps to lower it if needed. Remember, if you're serious about your health and that of your family, you'll need to work at reducing the sodium in your diet. If you really want to lower your family's sodium intake, eat less processed and restaurant / fast food, and more plant based natural Green Light foods! Refer to the Food Stop Light Chart for examples of these foods.

15
Sleep: Get your ZZZZZZs

Nowhere is it more obvious that we need a holistic approach to weight loss than when we consider sleep. The body is a complicated machine. We still have much to learn about how all of our body's systems work in concert to affect our overall health. During my Navy career, I experienced how the body reacts to working around the clock, the lack of sleep, and crushing stress. They all affect the body's overall well-being and even the ability to lose weight.

In the simplest terms, the body interprets the lack of sleep (tiredness) as the need for more calories. Our early ancestors' sleep patterns probably followed the cadence of the setting and rising sun. Without any artificial light (and no TV, Internet or smart phones) to keep them occupied, they probably slept more regularly and were better rested than 95 percent of us today.

Our ancestors probably got more sleep in the winter months due to there being less light. The longer days of summer brought less sleep and more than likely signaled their bodies to eat more in order to store fat for the winter. Your response to less sleep (hunger) is the result

> Many studies have shown that you'll eat more if you're sleep deprived.

of millions of years of human adaptation to the environment. While I wouldn't blame the obesity epidemic in America on our general lack of sleep, it is certainly a causal factor in our inability to achieve an appropriate weight for our height.

Many studies have shown that you'll eat more if you're sleep deprived. This is due to leptin* and other hormone level changes in your body when you get less sleep. I used to think that if

---

* Wikipedia: Leptin (Greek leptos meaning thin) is a 16 kDa protein hormone that plays a key role in regulating energy intake and energy expenditure, including appetite and metabolism.

I stayed up longer when I was trying to lose weight, I would burn more calories. Seemed to make sense, but the truth is that without sufficient sleep, leptin levels drop, signaling the body to eat.

If we are chronically sleep deprived, we always seem hungry, even after we eat, so we just eat all day long. Over time, as we gain significant weight, our body's can develop leptin resistance. When this happens, not only do we want to eat all the time, but the body thinks it is starving and you guessed it, it throttles back the calorie burn to survive. This is exactly opposite of what you want to do if you are trying to lose weight!

The picture of me in the tower of the USS Carl Vinson was taken during a period of my career when I got very little sleep. I sure don't look healthy in that photo and I can tell you I didn't lose any weight. In fact, during the 77 continuous days we fought the Afghanistan war, I averaged four hours of sleep per night. Not only was I a physical wreck when we headed home, but I had gained weight and it took me nearly a year to catch up on sleep. It was during this time and the beginning of my weight loss journey that I discovered the correlation between sleep and the body's ability to function appropriately to lose weight.

Recent studies of college students also reported that when they lacked sufficient sleep, their food choices steered toward junk or fast foods. The research couldn't determine if it was because they were too tired to prepare a healthy meal or if they just craved certain fast foods. It's probably a little of both, but I bet it's also due to the fact that the body craves quick energy and therefore we choose calorie-dense choices such as potato chips and cookies that provide a quick energy boost.

Without a full night's sleep, the hormone ghrelin* increases

---

* Wikipedia: Ghrelin is a hormone produced in the lining of the human stomach and epsilon cells of the pancreas that stimulate hunger. Ghrelin levels increase before meals and decrease after meals. It is considered the counterpart of the hormone leptin, which induces satiation when present at higher levels.

sending hunger signals to the body and can act in concert with your lower levels of leptin to increase appetite and torpedo your weight loss efforts the following day. When considering sleep, it's important to note how studies have also linked the hormone ghrelin with stress. Stress and the lack of sleep often occur at the same time.

While we can never eliminate all stress, how we handle it is key to our overall well-being. Obviously, the better physical shape you are in, the better you will be able to handle the normal stresses of this modern world. See the next chapter for more on handling stress.

Having experienced sustained, high-level stress, I was able to see how achieving an appropriate weight for my height, combined with exercise and a good night's sleep really helped me cope with stress. Eating well, getting sufficient sleep, and including a stress-relieving cardio workout will not only help you lose weight, it will help you deal with stress. Less stress = lower ghrelin = reduced hunger. It's eye opening when you see all the pieces start to fit together!

In my younger years of flying Navy jets I followed the shore liberty mantra "Eating is cheating, and you can sleep when you're dead." By the time I reached my mid-forties, I could see the negative effects this type of abuse had on my body. Today, I better understand how sleep and good nutrition positively contribute to my overall well-being. Bottom line: You need at least seven hours of sleep per night, eight if you can get it, especially during a weight loss journey.

> You need at least seven hours of sleep per night, eight if you can get it, especially during a weight loss journey.

16

Stress

Stress has been a normal part of the human condition for millions of years. Stress, and the body's reaction to it, is yet another example of how we humans developed a physiological response to help our bodies adapt to the environment. If a lion were chasing you across the Serengeti, your senses would be heightened, you would experience a much needed burst of energy, and your body would rapidly increase blood flow and metabolic rate. This is often referred to as the "fight or flight" response.

Fast-forward to today, and while we're not being chased across the Serengeti, many of us experience long periods of elevated stress due to our overloaded schedules. Not only are our bodies <u>not</u> well adapted to these long periods of stress, the connection between stress and weight gain is well established.

> The connection between stress and weight gain is well established.

A stress hormone called cortisol* is responsible for the body's rapid shift to the fight or flight response. Under normal conditions, this is a short-lived event and the body (after out-smarting that lion), slowly relaxes and returns to what is called homeostasis. If your body is unable to return to this relaxed condition, a host of bad things can happen to your body, such as increased belly fat and associated weight gain.

Most of us have seen the ads on TV hawking a supplement, disingenuously called *Cortislim* that claims it will magically make your belly fat disappear. As I've said, if these types of pills really worked, why isn't my doctor prescribing them for me?

---

* Wikipedia: Cortisol, also known as hydrocortisone, is a steroid hormone or glucocorticoid produced by the adrenal gland. It is released in response to stress.

The answer, of course, is obvious. They don't work! Just ask the folks who lost their money on this weight loss scheme and are now part of a class action suit.

Because you're reading this book and <u>not</u> trying to outsource your weight problem, you know better than to rely on TV commercials or the Internet for quick weight loss schemes. If you're one of the many Americans that experience elevated or prolonged stress in your daily life, you may not realize that it's more appropriate to use natural remedies to reduce your stress and return to homeostasis.

While this book's main focus is to help you lose weight, the same skills of eating better, exercising and getting sufficient sleep, will not only help you handle stress, but will also help you lead a less stressful life. Once you achieve an appropriate weight for your height, you'll have one less thing to be stressed-out about.

First of all, we need to identify the indicators of too much stress. Having just one indicator doesn't mean you're experiencing too much stress, but if you have several, it could mean you need to learn how to de-stress. In no particular order, the body's markers for stress are listed below. Having some of the symptoms will negatively affect your quality of life and will clearly impact your overall health, not to mention how they will impede your ability to lose weight.

<u>Markers for Stress</u> (in no particular order)

Anger	Anxiety
Irritability	Worry
Chest Pain	Muscle Tension
Depression	Sadness
High Blood Pressure	Exhaustion
Headache	Shortness of Breath
Restlessness	Decreased Libido

Job Dissatisfaction
Forgetfulness
Chest Pain
Sweating
Resentment
Guilt
Weight Gain
Diarrhea
Back Pain
Grinding Teeth
Abusing Alcohol
Burnout
Negative Attitude

Insecurity
Inability to Concentrate
Mood Swings
Confusion
Sleep Problems
Skin Breakouts
Constipation
Upset Stomach
Clenched Jaws
Frequent Illness
Emotional Eating
Neck Pain

How we deal with stress will affect our ability to achieve an appropriate weight for our height.

Here are some strategies that worked for me:

1. **<u>Remove the things that cause you stress</u>**. Now I'm not suggesting you shoot your boss, but there are other ways to remove some of the stress in your life. For example, if that funny sound that your car makes has you fretting the entire way to work every day, perhaps you should drop your car off at the repair shop on your way to work tomorrow.

2. **<u>Avoid stressful situations</u>**. This doesn't mean putting off your dentist appointment, but if you can arrange your schedule so you can leave for work 15 minutes earlier to avoid that traffic jam every workday, then do it.

3. **<u>Set realistic goals and then prioritize them</u>**. Every morning at work, I write down all the things I need to do that day and quickly realize it's twice as much as I realistically can accomplish. This used to be stressful for me, so now I prioritize the top three and work to just

complete them. Many of the items on the original list make it to the top three within a couple of days and I now realize those that don't, really aren't that important.

4. **Learn to take a break and relax**. Don't go out for a smoke, but go outside and walk around the building or block just once. You'll feel the sun on your face, smell the fresh air and come back inside feeling a whole lot better.

5. **Exercise**. If you're fortunate like me, you can use a gym during the workday. If not, hit the gym or get some exercise before or after work. This is one of the very best ways to relieve stress and get the calories burning!

6. **Re-evaluate how you are reacting to someone or viewing a certain situation**. Try to see at least some element of an alternative viewpoint. Ask yourself if you are overreacting. Achieving some small element of common ground with a troublesome co-worker can really reduce the stress level at work.

7. **Learn to unwind once you get home**. I found that I needed to establish a sanctuary where I can go after our family dinner to unwind before bedtime. My wife knows she is invited, but that this isn't the time to talk. The original plans for our house called this space "the quiet room" and that is exactly what I use it for. Abusing drugs or alcohol is obviously the wrong way to "unwind."

8. **Sleep**. A full night's restorative sleep (7-8 hours) does wonders for your perspective the next day and helps keep those important hormones in balance.

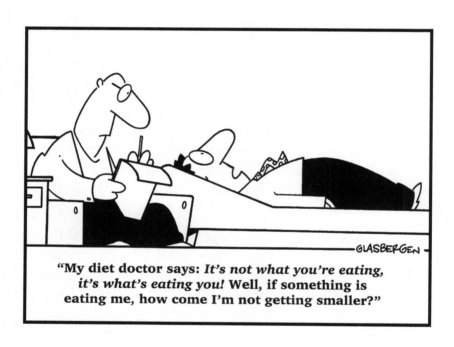

"My diet doctor says: *It's not what you're eating, it's what's eating you!* Well, if something is eating me, how come I'm not getting smaller?"

17
What Should I Weigh?

When asked how tall a man should be, Abraham Lincoln once said, "A man should be tall enough so his feet reach the ground." Many people want to know the answer to the question, "How much should I weigh?" In this metric-obsessed world, we want to quickly calculate the possibilities and the necessary effort / willingness to go from our current weight to a hopefully reasonable and achievable goal.

Unfortunately, my Lincoln-like answer to the question, "How much should I weigh?" is generally, "Less than you think." If you've already looked at the Target Weight Chart at the end of this chapter, you know why I'm saying this.

> I discovered that humans are not designed to gain weight throughout their adult life.

This was the question that I asked myself, repeatedly, early in my journey. Believe it or not, it was some time before I realized that I should probably weigh what I did when I was in the best shape of my life, as I explained in Chapter 10.

I discovered that humans are not designed to gain weight throughout their adult life. I thought gaining weight was a normal part of the aging process. However, we humans gain weight as adults mostly because we never get rid of that fat we store for the winter, along with a high calorie diet and little exercise.

> Ideally, most of us should maintain the weight we achieve in our late teens and early twenties.

Ideally, most of us should maintain the weight we achieve in our late teens and early twenties. That's a scary thought, especially for me since I was 148 pounds throughout my teens and early twenties. I reached the high 160s only after I added some muscle mass due to the Navy exercise program. If my late teen height and weight of 5' 11" and 148 pounds seem impossibly skinny (or even sickly), I'll note that I had a BMI of nearly 21, still well within a healthy weight range for someone of my height. I'll also note that this same skinny kid was 55 pounds heavier a little more than 28 years later (148 lbs + 55 lbs = 203 lbs).

I realize that understanding what you should weigh can be very discouraging. Here's the good news: For every few pounds you lose to get closer to your target weight, you markedly reduce your potential for cancer and others diseases, as well as improve the quality of your life and potential for longevity. How much you want to lose depends on you, which is why I say it's a journey and not a time-bound diet. My weight loss journey is in its seventh year.

> Don't confuse the word "diet," defined as "what a person eats," for the act of losing weight, commonly and incorrectly described as "dieting."

Even though I long ago achieved an appropriate weight for my height, I continue to learn and refine my diet. Don't confuse the word "diet," defined as "what a person eats," for the act of losing weight, commonly and incorrectly described as "dieting." For many of us, addressing our diet will help us achieve an appropriate weight for our height through weight loss. That's the correct way to think about it. I'm successful because I'm engaged in a thought process about what it takes to achieve and maintain a healthy weight.

But you still want to know what you should weigh. The Target Weight Chart may seem ridiculously out of whack. Most people say there is no way they could ever weigh their optimum weight according to this chart. I generally go through the, "what did you weigh in high school / when you got married drill," and invariably, their weight then was very close to the Target Weight Chart.

Now if you looked like Arnold Schwarzenegger when he was Mr. Olympia, clearly you'll be off the chart. That's why I include a body fat range for both men and woman. Your local gym, personal trainer or doctor can easily measure your body fat. Mine is 14.8 percent.

I combined information from several sources for the Target Weight Chart. It includes the age-old nutritionist standard for both men and women, the maximum weight recommendations from the National Diabetes Education Program (NDEP), the current Navy standards, and the height / weight associated with a BMI in the 21-24 range. The numbers on the chart are median weights and depending on your frame size, you could easily be at a healthy weight within 10 pounds either way of the listed weight.

There was absolutely nothing I could find to indicate we can be much heavier and still be healthy. There have been various studies over time that concluded overweight people live longer or they are as healthy, or healthier, than folks at an appropriate weight for their height. But you really have to read these studies carefully to understand the relevance.

It is possible to be overweight and have very normal blood pressure and cholesterol readings, especially in your 40s and 50s. What many people don't realize is that these overweight individuals may be healthy right up until their doctor tells them they have cancer or heart disease, ultimately shaving 10-15 years off their normal lifespan. Those few overweight people that live into their 70s and 80s often have so many ailments that their quality of life just isn't very good. The choice is ours to make.

> My recommendation is to view the target weight associated with your height as an ultimate (stretch) goal.

My recommendation is to view the target weight associated with your height as an ultimate (stretch) goal. If the chart indicates you're obese, your first goal should be to achieve a BMI of less than 30. It'll surprise you how many "normal" looking people are classified as obese. Then aim for a BMI of 25 and below. Once you've made it that far you'll have the knowledge and understanding of what practices you must continue to achieve your optimum weight.

> I'm challenged on my height / weight chart more than anything else I say in my weight loss seminars.

It's okay if you take two years to lose 80 pounds. When you think about, if it takes you 34 weeks to reach your goal (as I did), the chances of you going back to your old weight are less likely. If you learn what it takes to lose weight consistently over that length of time, you've really broken the code on permanent weight loss. That's why Basic Truth #2 is so important, and why quick weight-loss schemes will never be able to deliver <u>permanent</u> weight loss. Remember, that's your goal!

If you get started and don't see immediate results, remember, at least you're not gaining weight. For so many of us the simple act of no longer gaining weight over a period of weeks / months is an enormous victory. If the chart says you need to lose 40 pounds and you only lose 20 in the next year, you have significantly reduced your incidence for disease and have done wonders for your longevity and future quality of life.

I'm challenged on my height / weight chart more than anything else I say in my weight loss seminars. People say the chart shows ridiculously low weights and that there is no way they'll ever achieve those weights. My response is that I cannot find anything that indicates we should be heavier than those weights.

If you are very muscular (which most of us are not), you'll be way over the weight listed for your height so simply shoot for the body fat percentages (13-17 percent for men, 19-23 percent for women). The mistake we make is that we compare ourselves to those around us. In America today, fully two-thirds of us are either overweight or obese. It's our perspective that needs to change along with our waistline (a maximum 40 inches for men, 35 for women).

It's our perspective that needs to change along with our waistline (a maximum 40 inches for men, 35 for women).

In the book *Flyboys*, James Bradley describes the height and weight of several of the Chichi Jima aviators when they joined the Navy. I was amazed at how different the body composition was for naval aviators back in the 1940s. These pilots and aircrews flew the TBM Avenger, the F4U Corsair and the SB2C dive-bomber. You had to be healthy and strong to fly those rugged machines and withstand the G-forces those aircraft were capable of producing.

These men were not wimps. In fact, they were the best physical specimens of their day, yet consider their height and weights: 5'7" / 128 lbs (Ensign Floyd Hall); 5'9" / 129 lbs (Petty Officer Third Class, Marve Mershon); and 6' / 169 lbs (Aviation Radioman Second Class, Lloyd Woellhof).

Don't those heights and weights seem unbelievably skinny by today's standards and even compared with my chart? Yet those WWII aviators are much more in line with what our ancestors weighed than what we weigh today. This is true even when we compare the *Flyboy* aviators to the young men and women flying our comparable jets today. It shows you how far out of balance we have become in the United States and why we have so many health concerns.

In addition to seeing your target weight on the next page, check out the BMI Chart on page 170 to calculate your Body Mass Index. By following these two measures, you can set the goals for your weight loss journey.

In addition to seeing your target weight on the next page, check out the BMI Chart in the back of the book to calculate your Body Mass Index.

Target Weight for Your Height Chart

Height in inches	Males	Females	Height in inches	Males	Females
60"	118	110	69"	158	148
61"	122	114	70"	163	152
62"	126	118	71"	168	156
63"	130	122	72"	173	160
64"	134	126	73"	178	164
65"	138	130	74"	184	168
66"	143	134	75"	190	173
67"	147	139	76"	195	178
68"	152	143			

Heavily muscled individuals should
have body fat measurements taken.
Men's body fat = 13-17% • Women's body fat = 19-23%

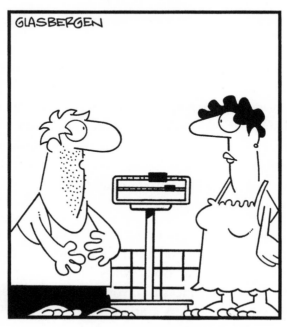

"The reason for my weight gain is
obvious — humans are evolving
into a larger species!"

18

All Fats Are Not Created Equal

The human body needs fat. You need fat to survive, so you must have some fat in your diet. Knowing how much fat, what types, and where they come from are critical to good health and achieving an appropriate weight for your height. You need to understand that the calories from all types of fat are the same, about 120 calories per tablespoon. The fats you <u>choose</u> will make a lot of difference in your health.

> Knowing how much fat, what types, and where they come from are critical to good health and achieving an appropriate weight for your height.

Our doctors have told many of us to reduce the fat in our diet, more than likely because our body has stored more fat than is healthy for us. What they don't generally have time to tell us is which fats to avoid, which foods contain bad fats, and which fats are good for us.

Many recently published studies tracked folks who reduced the fat in their diet to see if this had an effect on their overall health. Most of the studies didn't differentiate between the so-called good and bad fats. Many directed the participants to reduce the fat in their diet by 10-25 percent, but didn't track what kinds of fat they consumed. The results, not surprisingly, were not that impressive and clearly didn't provide useful information about which fats are most harmful.

After learning about the different fats and adjusting my diet, I changed my lipid (cholesterol) profile remarkably. My total cholesterol number went down from 273 to 167. My HDLs (high density lipoproteins), the good type of cholesterol, changed from a not-so-good 35 to a much healthier 80. An HDL number

To raise your HDL (good) cholesterol, exercise more. To lower your LDL (bad) cholesterol, improve your diet.

of 60 or above is generally considered to provide protection against heart disease.

My LDL (low density lipoproteins), the bad cholesterol, changed from 188 to 95, which is great since doctors these days like to see LDLs below 100 (some even say below 90). My triglycerides (fat in the blood) changed from 157 to 37. Your doctor will want your triglyceride level to be below 150. The best way to lower your triglycerides is, you guessed it, to lose weight. To raise your HDL (good) cholesterol, exercise more. To lower your LDL (bad) cholesterol, improve your diet.

I made these changes through a combination of diet, exercise and 20 mg of a prescription drug called *Zocor* each day. Hey, that's what the commercials on TV tell us to do. Amazing! If you listen to the cholesterol medication commercials on TV they always say "when diet and exercise are not enough" indicating that you should combine the medication with both improved diet and exercise. I was already exercising regularly, so it was the diet part that was most important for me. I'm here to tell you that this combination works!

Worst to Best Types of Fat

Types of Fats

There are five basic types of fats. From **worst to best** they are: trans fat, saturated fat, unsaturated fat, omega-6 fatty acids and omega-3 fatty acids.

Absolute Worst

1. **Trans fat** is the absolute worst type of fat because our bodies have had so little time to adapt to it. It's only existed for 40 years or so. Trans fat is created when

manufacturers add hydrogen to vegetable oils during a process called hydrogenation. Our HDLs have a hard time scrubbing these fats out of our arteries, thereby markedly increasing our chances for heart attack and stroke.

Trans fat is found mostly in baked goods, stick margarine, solid shortening and fried foods, but it's also in many foods you may not suspect. Most peanut butter has a little trans fat, as do some breakfast cereals. Your goal should be to have zero trans fat in your diet.

The problem with trans fat is that it is so insidious. It's in foods you eat without knowing it. Recent press reports indicate that the public is becoming more aware of trans fat and demanding that it be removed from restaurant fare (where there are generally no food labels to indicate how much trans fat you're getting). Be careful and consider asking your server about the ingredients if you want to avoid trans fats.

The FDA has allowed manufacturers to state "0 grams of trans fat per serving" when a serving contains less than one gram of trans fat. In foods that are fairly dependent on trans fat, the manufacturers have simply reduced the serving size so the trans fat is just less than one gram. You're probably eating four to five of the recommended servings and getting three-four grams of trans fat. *I Can't Believe It's Not Butter Spray* is one of these types of foods.

You have to look for the words "hydrogenated " or "partially hydrogenated" in the list of ingredients to know if the product has any trans fat, potentially a fair amount of it, even if the label says "0 grams of trans fat per serving". *I Can't Believe It's Not Butter Spray* legally states that it has "No trans fat, per serving" because the trans fats in a single serving (5 sprays / 1 gram) contains less than one gram of trans fat. The font size of "0g trans fat" is very large compared to the "per serving" information.

Just to put the serving size in perspective, each spray container has 226 individual servings (1130 sprays). That means a single bottle would last you 226 individual meals. That's clearly not reasonable for most people. If you use this spray, I guarantee you're getting more trans fat than you ever imagined.

The information on the *I Can't Believe It's Not Butter* (and other food manufacturers') web sites is very misleading as well. You'll see how easy it is to construe that you're not consuming any trans fat, or calories for that matter. I know people that pour (not spray) *I Can't Believe It's Not Butter* on their vegetables without knowing that it does in fact have calories, saturated and trans fat (although the label claims "zero" for all three). This is an example of what you're up against! Educating yourself is the key. See Chapter 23 for more guidance on deciphering food labels.

Bad

2. **Saturated fat**, the most common fat in today's food supply, comes mostly from animals. Some common animal-based saturated fat foods include steak, ribs, bacon, hot dogs, bratwurst, butter, sour cream, milk, ice cream, cheese, chicken (especially the skin), and lunch meats. Some saturated fats come from foods cooked in animal fats, such as potato chips. These foods not only provide us with unwanted saturated fat, they are also very calorie-dense.

    Saturated fat raises your bad cholesterol (LDL) and puts you at risk for heart disease (heart attack and stroke). You can tell if it's saturated fat because it's hard at room temperature. Check out that leftover gravy when you take it out of the refrigerator. Again, I repeat: To lower your bad cholesterol, reduce the saturated and trans fat foods in your diet. To raise your good cholesterol (HDL), increase the amount of exercise you get.

Your doctor may also prescribe statin drugs (*Lipitor*, *Crestor*, *Zocor*, etc.) that could also positively affect these numbers. But keep in mind that they must be combined with a healthy low-fat diet and exercise for best results. I saw this correlation during my weight loss journey and was able to dramatically improve both numbers.

Somewhat Better

3. **Unsaturated fat** is the type of fat that comes from plants. This includes both **monounsaturated** and **polyunsaturated** fats. Your body is well adapted to these fats since humans have been eating them for millions of years. Unfortunately, the calories in unsaturated fats are just as high as those in saturated fats. So while you are well adapted to them, remember that the calories still count!

   Common **monounsaturated** fat foods include avocados (which are very good for you since they help your body absorb nutrients), olive oil, most nuts, and oils made from nuts such as canola and peanut. Polyunsaturated fat is found in oil from seeds including corn, safflower, sesame, soybean and sunflower. Many margarines contain both poly and monounsaturated fats.

Better

4. **Omega-6** fatty acid is also a polyunsaturated fat that belongs to a family of fats called "essential fatty acids." Without getting too technical, the problem with our diet today in America is that we get too many omega-6 fats

and not enough omega-3s. **Omega-6 fats are many of the oils in processed foods,** including safflower, sunflower, corn, sesame and soybean. During the past 60 years, our intake of omega-6 fats has doubled while omega-3s have dropped to one-sixth of what our prairie-inhabiting ancestors got back in the 1850s.

A healthy diet should have omega-6 and omega-3 fatty acids in a ratio of about 3:1 (three omega-6 to one omega-3). Many Americans have diets that fall in the range of 20:1 omega-6 to omega-3. Too much omega-6 fat in your diet **may** lead to water retention, raised blood pressure and increased blood clotting. **To lower your intake of omega-6 fatty acids, reduce the amount of processed food in your diet.** It can get very confusing. For example, soybeans contain healthy omega-3 fats, while soybean oil has the omega-6 fats we should all try to reduce.

Many vegetables also contain the good omega-3 fats, including spinach, kale, Brussels sprouts, broccoli, spring greens and any dark lettuce leaves. Not surprisingly, these are all foods you should eat, which I call Green Light foods. I explain them in the next chapters along with the Food Stoplight Charts.

Best

5. <u>**Omega-3 fatty acids**</u> are the so-called good fats. The "Mediterranean diet," rich in these types of fat, has been shown to influence many of the factors that protect you from cardiovascular disease. What foods are in the Mediterranean diet? Fish, especially salmon, herring, mackerel and rainbow trout, as well as soybeans, butternut and winter squash, flax (seed and oil), walnuts, olive oil and canola oil. Omega-3 fats may help regulate blood

sugar levels, increase metabolic rate (helping weight loss), and aide in the prevention of diabetes and obesity.

Studies have linked increased omega-3 intake (fatty fish five times a week) to a decrease in certain types of strokes in women. Several studies have shown that increased omega-3 in the diet may improve cognitive function. One study indicated that the average 100 grams per day of fatty fish that Japanese men consumed protected their hearts and dramatically lowered their incidence of heart attacks, in spite of their reputation as heavy smokers and drinkers.

This is about as technical as this book gets (my brain hurts already). <u>Remember that the calories are the same for all fats at about 120 calories per tablespoon.</u> The bottom line is that you should develop a diet that provides no more than 20-25% of your daily calories from fat, and most of them should be the omega-3 and omega-6 poly and monounsaturated fats, versus trans and saturated fats.

See Chapter 25, By the Numbers, that outlines the government's (and my) recommendations for daily consumption. Eat a diet that includes green vegetables and fish. It's the right way to eat because that's the way our ancestors ate for millions of years.

19

Calorie Density: Eat More, Weigh Less

It may seem counterintuitive, but you really can eat more to weigh less. I realize this may sound like so many of the ridiculous ads we see on TV and hear on the radio that claim effortless weight loss. While eating more to weigh less isn't effortless, and you certainly can't do it with cheeseburgers and pizza, it's definitely doable if you manage your calorie density.

You'll recall from Chapter 10 where I stated there is only one way to lose weight: Consume fewer calories than you burn. This is still true! You'll also remember Basic Truth #1 states that to lose weight we can't be hungry and we still must eat and enjoy our food.

With a little planning, you can eat more than enough food every day to stay satisfied, energized and still lose weight. Calorie density is the key. The calorie density of foods influences your hunger, satiety and food intake. For example, a dinner salad with dressing may have about 100 calories while a small square of chocolate may have the same number. But the former will help fill you while the latter will just make you crave more. By eating foods with lower calorie density, you will feel fuller but have eaten fewer calories.

So what is calorie density? This is where a little science goes a long way. The calorie density (or energy density) of a food is a measurement of the average calories per weight (gram or ounce) of that food. The biggest factor in determining calorie density is the water content of a food. Water increases the volume of a food without adding calories. Volume is important for feeling like you've eaten enough to feel full or satisfied. Obviously, the foods with more volume and fewer calories will be your best choices.

You can use calorie density to compare the number of calories in equal amounts of different foods and make better food choices. For example, one ounce of chocolate has far more calories (i.e. a higher calorie density) than one ounce of pretzels. This means that if you eat one ounce of chocolate you will consume more calories than if you eat one ounce of pretzels. Pretzels have a lower calorie density and are therefore a better choice when counting calories (although pretzels are mostly refined grains).

> Calorie density (CD) is calculated as the amount of calories contained in one gram of a given food.

Calorie density (CD) is calculated as the amount of calories contained in one gram of a given food. For example, 100 grams of spinach has 23 calories. This means that one gram of spinach contains 0.23 calories. Therefore the CD of spinach is 0.23. In general, calorie density is categorized from very low = 0.00 to 0.7; low to moderate = 0.8 to 1.5; moderate to high = 1.6 to 3.0, and very high = 3.1 and above. The calorie densities of a few foods are listed below.

<u>Calorie Density (CD)</u> (per gram of food)

Cucumbers - 0.13	Apple – 0.58
Tuna – 1.2	Cheese – 4.1
Tomatoes - 0.21	Grapes – 0.67
Turkey – 1.7	Bacon - 5.0
Broccoli - 0.28	Green Beans – 0.78
Salmon – 2.1	Chocolate – 5.4
Grapefruit - 0.30	Corn – 0.86
Big Mac – 2.5	Peanut Butter – 5.9
Watermelon - 0.32	Banana – 0.92
Bread – 2.6.	Butter – 7.2
Carrots - 0.43	Shrimp – 1.0
French Fries – 3	Mayonnaise – 7.2
Blueberries - 0.56	Sweet Potato – 1.0
Pretzels – 3.9	Olive Oil – 8.9

It's important to understand that we're preprogrammed to want the most calorie-dense foods. The problem these days is threefold. First, our early ancestors sought the most calorie-dense foods since any excess calories would be stored as fat for times when the food supply got scarce. We still have this deeply rooted desire for calories, so when we have a choice, we tend to choose calorie-dense foods.

The second problem is that our cash-strapped wallets are helping us make these same bad choices. The refined grain, fat, sugar and high fructose corn syrup-laden foods are both cheaper and are more available than fresh foods due to their longer shelf life. Finally, our lifestyles are more sedentary, often with little or no exercise, but our pre-programmed desire for calorie-laden foods has not abated.

> We're preprogrammed to want the most calorie-dense foods.

Understanding how we are preprogrammed, we now know why "thinking is not necessary" weight loss programs are destined to fail. In my case, I had to train myself to choose foods I both liked and enjoyed, but that were low or lower, calorie-dense than I otherwise would have chosen.

I mentioned previously that I introduced Dr Pratt's *superfoods* into my diet and was amazed at the results. I was still eating the same amount, or volume, of food each day, but it contained fewer calories. As a "What" eater, I didn't change my workout routine (calories burned each day), but changed the number of calories I was consuming.

I could have tried to eat the same foods by adjusting the amount / size so the calories would have been more in line with what I burned each day. For example, I could have chosen a single burger, small fries and a small soft drink at one of the many fast food restaurants near my place of work. This, of course, would have violated Basic Truth #1 as I undoubtedly still would have been hungry.

Instead, I chose a lean protein (low-sodium turkey slices) or a few mixed nuts, an 80-calorie non-fat yogurt, a bag of grapes and a diet soda. Nowadays, I just choose water with that meal and I'm quite satiated. In addition, I've managed my blood sugar, maintained energy until dinner time, and consumed fewer calories than if I'd chosen the smallest portions at the local burger joint. This is an example of applying calorie density in a weight loss journey.

Many people at my seminars say, "I can't learn to eat this way." I too believed that when I started. But when I discovered that I really enjoyed many (but not all) of the foods that were fairly low in calorie density, I changed my thinking. The fat, salt and sugar in our processed foods act the same way as illegal drugs. We need ever-increasing amounts to stay satisfied because our tongues have become deadened to the taste. The food manufacturers know this and they keep supplying us with ever-increasing amounts of fats, salt and sugar to keep our taste buds interested.

I succeeded in revamping my diet because I had two things going for me. First, I was engaged in the process. Second, by trying various low calorie-dense foods I found the ones I really liked. I still had the five million years of genetic programming steering me towards cheeseburgers, but I had learned to listen to my body. I realized that plant-based, low calorie foods made me feel better. They also provided me with more energy and greater stamina.

As I mentioned earlier, you probably eat about the same volume of food each day. Eating foods that are low calorie, and make you feel full, can really help keep your calorie intake in line with your calorie output. I often include a bag full of grapes in my lunch because they're delicious and really satisfy my hunger. I can feel how heavy it is by just holding the bag and not surprisingly, it really fills me up without driving up my calorie intake for the day.

See the Green Light Foods chart on page 107 for a full listing of low calorie-dense foods. As you include those Green Light foods in your diet, you'll start to feel better and lose weight. Here's what 200 calories of two of my favorite foods look like. That's 740 grams of mini-peppers and 290 grams of grapes, each one only at 200 calories. Water-dense foods such as grapes and mini-peppers are low calorie-dense and when combined with whole grains and lean protein, can really help you feel full.

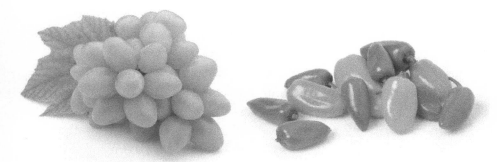

You'll remember Barry Popkin from Chapter 11 who taught us we have separate thirst and hunger mechanisms. It seems that when we eat high water content food, instead of just drinking water (which is still important), the water in the food stays in our stomachs longer and adds to that satisfied feeling of being full. You may see this defined as satiety.

The bottom line is that most of us should consciously eat more low-calorie foods for both good health and weight loss. The hard part is choosing the apple and grapes over the cheeseburger and fries. Sure your favorite fast food restaurant has some healthy choices, but can you override five million years of genetic coding and buy the apple and yogurt when your nostrils are filled with the scent of a *Big Mac*? I can't! That's why I bring my lunch with me and rarely venture out to the fast food establishments with my coworkers at lunchtime. It takes that kind

> The bottom line is that most of us should consciously eat more low-calorie foods for both good health and weight loss.

of <u>commitment</u> to avoid high-calorie comfort food or super-human willpower, which few of us have.

Many people tell me that they could never eat like me and seemed discouraged when I explain what I eat in a normal day. What I tell them is that they were designed to eat just like I do. Sure, at first it seems daunting to change from your current diet to the low calorie, plant based diet that will help you lose weight and return you to good health. Remember, I changed my diet over months and years, but only to foods that I really enjoyed eating. When I saw that I was losing weight and had so much more energy, the changes became easier.

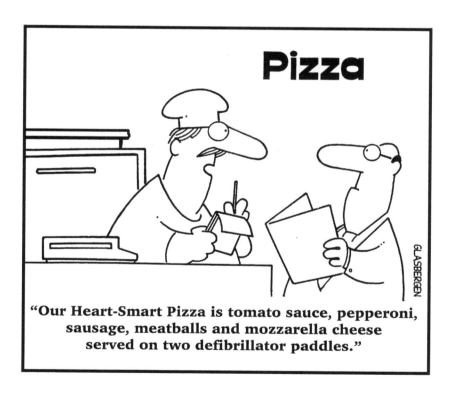

"Our Heart-Smart Pizza is tomato sauce, pepperoni, sausage, meatballs and mozzarella cheese served on two defibrillator paddles."

A Day of Ed's Meals

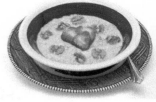

Breakfast

- Seasonal fruit – grapefruit in the winter and strawberries, blueberries, melon, cantaloupe, etc. fruit in season

- *Cheerios* or *Nature's Path Organic Flax Plus Granola with Pumpkin Seed* cereal with fat-free milk

- Black coffee

Lunch

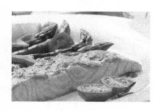

- Mini-peppers, carrots or any other easily transportable vegetable

- Seasonal fresh fruit (apples, orange, plums, pears, etc)

- Handful of mixed nuts or *Planters NUT-trition* smoked almonds

- *Dannon, Light & Fit* 80-calorie yogurt

Dinner

- Chicken or fish most nights of the week, prepared simply. Favorite is salmon with *Grey Poupon Country* or any coarse ground mustard spread over the fillet, then baked or grilled on a cedar plank.

- Once a week, red meat, either steak (NY strip) or lamb chops. Cook lamp chops in an uncovered deep frying pan, with olive oil and fresh rosemary.

- Spaghetti with low-sodium tomato sauce (sometimes with sweet Italian sausage)

- Steamed vegetables – favorites are green beans, broccoli, Brussels sprouts and carrots

- Tomatoes – sliced thin with a drizzle of balsamic vinegar and olive oil, fresh basil, garlic powder and a sprinkle of feta cheese

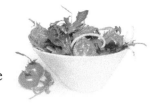

- Wine (mostly red)

- Dark chocolate (at least 60% cacao), occasionally *Edy's Slow Churned (Light) Vanilla* ice cream

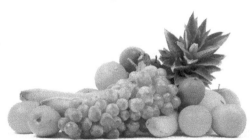

Snacks

- Fruit

- *Triscuit* (whole grain / rye) with natural peanut butter

- Mixed nuts

- Smoked salmon

20

The Food Stoplight Charts

The charts in this chapter are a helpful resource for everyone, but "What" eaters should find them particularly useful. They'll help you choose foods that are delicious, good for you, and generally lower in calories than many of the foods you're eating now.

Using the charts is easy. Green Light foods are the absolute best for you and should be a major part of your diet. They represent very low-calorie foods. Yellow Light foods are not bad for you per se. You can enjoy them carefully as the calorie count really starts to go up. They're mostly medium calorie-dense foods.

Red Light foods can only be enjoyed "occasionally" since these foods contain significant calories and often also have artery-clogging fats. These are your highest calorie foods and need to be avoided during a weight loss journey since they won't help you achieve that 500 calorie per day deficit. You can dip into the Red Light foods every once in a while after you have reached an appropriate weight for your height by consuming as many calories as you burn each day.

As a guide, your breakfast and lunch should mostly be Green Light foods. For breakfast, I combine seasonal fresh fruit with whole grain cereal and fat free milk and drink either black coffee or a latte with skim milk. For lunch, I pack a combination of fruit (grapes, apple, peach, blueberries), veggies (sweet peppers, raw carrots), protein (a small handful of nuts) and dairy (yogurt).

There are literally a million combinations, all from the Green Light Chart. Dinner is when I occasionally dip into the Yellow and Red Light categories. While I'll mostly choose either fish or chicken with steamed vegetables, whole wheat bread and red wine, once a week we have spaghetti or ravioli with a single steamed vegetable, and red meat (steak, lamb chops) on weekends.

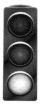

Green Light Foods:

Note: Dr. Pratt's *Superfoods* are listed in bold italics.

Almonds	***Apples***	Apricots
Artichokes	Asparagus	***Avocados***
Bananas	Barley	Beets
Beans*	***Blueberries***	Bran
Bread /Bagels / English Muffins (100% whole wheat)	***Broccoli***	Brussels sprouts
Cabbage (red / green)	Cantaloupe	Carrots
Cashews	Catfish	Cauliflower
Celery	Cereal (whole grain)	Cherries
Chick peas (hummus)	Chicken (white meat)	Chicken broth (low sodium)
Cinnamon	Clams	Cod
Coffee (black)	Collard greens	Corn
Cottage cheese (low fat)	Cranberry Juice (lite)	Cucumbers
Egg (whites)	Eggplant	Endamame
Flounder	***Garlic***	Grapes
Grapefruit	Green Beans	Halibut
Kale	***Kiwi***	Kumquats

* Beans include green, lima, pinto, black, butter, string, garbanzo (Chick peas), black, kidney, navy, white, lentils and waxed

Lemons	Lentils	Lettuce
Mackerel	Mangoes	Melon
Milk (fat free)	Monkfish	Mushrooms
Mustard	Nectarines	***Oats / Oatmeal***
Okra	***Olive oil***	***Onions***
Oranges	Papayas	Pasta (whole wheat)
Peaches	Peanuts	Pears
Peas	Pecans	Peppers
Persimmons	Pickles	Pistachios
Plums	***Pomegranates***	***Pumpkin***
Prunes	Quinoa	Radishes
Raisins	Raspberries	Relish (sweet)
Rice (brown)	Rockfish	***Salmon***
Salsa	Sardines	Sauerkraut
Shredded wheat	Shrimp (shellfish)	Snapper
Sole	***Soy***	***Spinach***
Squash	Strawberries	Sweet Potato
Swiss chard	Swordfish	Tangerines
Tilapia	***Tea***	Tofu
Tomatoes	Tomato sauce (low sodium)	Trout
Turkey (breast)	Turnip greens	Tuna
Veggie Burgers	Vegetable Juice (low salt)	Water
Watermelon	Walnuts	Yams
Yogurt (low fat)	Zucchini	

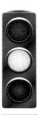

Yellow Light Foods:

Note: Dr. Pratt's *Superfoods* are listed in bold italics.

Applesauce	Bread / Bagels / English Muffins (multi grain)	Baked Potato
Baked Beans	Beef eye of round	Bran Flakes
Canola oil	Chicken (dark meat / livers)	***Chocolate (dark)***
Coconut	Crackers (whole grain)	Cream of wheat
Dates	Eggs (whole)	Fillet Mignon
Fruit Juice	Fruit (candied)	Granola
Granola Bar	Grits	***Honey***
Jell-O	Jelly and Jam	Lasagna (vegetable)
Latte (fat free milk)	London Broil	Margarine (low fat)
Milk (2%)	Mushrooms	New York Strip
Nuts	Olives	Orange juice
Oysters (raw)	Pancakes (whole wheat / buckwheat)	Pasta (refined grain)
Peanut Butter	Peanut oil	Pineapple
Pizza (cheese / whole wheat crust)	Popcorn (no butter)	Pork loin
Potatoes	Pretzels	Rice (white)
Saffron oil	Salad dressing (low fat)	Scallops
Soup (non-creamy)	Soybeans	Soymilk
Steak (lean cut)	Veal	Wine (red / white)

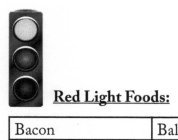

Red Light Foods:

Bacon	Baloney	Beef (ground)
Beer	Biscuits & gravy	Bratwurst
Bread (white)	Breakfast shakes	Brownies
Butter	Caesar salad	Cake
Canadian bacon	Candy	Cereal (sugared)
Cheese	Cheeseburger	Cheese cake
Chef's salad	Chicken salad	Chicken pot pie
Chicken wings	Chili	Chinese food
Chow mein	Cinnamon buns	Coffee cake
Cookies	Cornbread	Corn chips
Crackers	Cream cheese	Creamed Vegetables
Creamy salad dressing	Croissant	Croutons
Custard	Danish	Doughnuts
Duck	Eggnog	Enchiladas
Fish sticks	French fries	Fruitcake
Gravy	Grilled cheese	Half & Half (cream)
Ham	Hamburger	Hot dogs
Ice cream	Jelly beans	Lamb chops / roast
Lasagna (meat)	Lunchmeat	Macaroni & cheese
Macaroni salad	Marshmallows	Maple syrup
Mayonnaise	Meat loaf	Meatballs
Meatball sub	Mexican food	Milk (whole)
Milk chocolate	Milkshakes	Muffins

Nachos	Non-dairy creamer	Onion rings
Pastries	Philly cheese steak	Pies / Pie crust
Pizza (meat)	Pork chops	Pot pies
Potatoes au gratin	Potato chips	Potato salad
Potato / Pizza skins	Pudding	Quesadillas
Refried beans	Ribs (BBQ)	Rib Eye
Roast beef	Salad / Cooking oil	Salami
Saltines	Sausage	Scone
Sherbet	Snack cakes	Soda (sugared)
Sour cream	Soup (creamy)	Spaghetti with meat sauce
Sports drinks	Tacos	Taco salad
Tartar sauce	Tater tots	Toaster Pastries
Tuna melt	Tuna salad	Vanilla wafers
Veal cutlet	Venison	Vegetables with cheese
Vienna sausage	Waffles	Whipped cream

21

Glycemic Index

Several years ago, the commercial weight loss world realized that the glycemic index would be a great tool to market weight loss plans. In typical fashion, many of the "I don't want to think about weight loss" programs rolled out diets focused on "managing your glycemic index." It was the right idea, but the wrong execution. Not that any of these programs really wanted to educate us about the glycemic index, because if they did, we'd realize we don't need anything they are selling.

Here's what you need to know:

> Every food you eat has a glycemic index or a measure of how that food affects your blood sugar.

Every food you eat has a glycemic index or a measure of how that food affects your blood sugar. To be more precise, it is really the glycemic load (a combination of a food's glycemic index and total amount of carbohydrates eaten) that we should be concerned about. The glycemic index is simply a value that lets us know the quality of the carbohydrates (carbs) we are eating, not the quantity, and certainly not the calorie content. Understanding how individual foods can affect your blood sugar level is not only critical information for diabetics, it is also important for those of us who want to lose weight.

In the most basic terms, carbs are either simple or complex. Simple carbs are considered "bad" because they can cause a rapid rise in blood sugar. This is bad because after an initial spike, blood sugar plummets, causing us to feel tired and hungry. Complex carbs are considered "good" because when eaten in combination with other healthy foods, can help steady blood sugar levels and keep us satisfied (not hungry) longer. For example, white bread made with refined grains is bad, while whole wheat bread made with complex whole grains is good.

As I said, this is a gross oversimplification because the body's response to different complex carbs can vary widely. For example, watermelon has a high glycemic index but has a relatively low glycemic load because of its low carb count. This is just one example of the much misunderstood and commercially misused "glycemic index."

> The glycemic index (GI) is simply a measure of how quickly a particular food will turn into glucose (sugar) once it is eaten.

The glycemic index (GI) is simply a measure of how quickly a particular food will turn into glucose (sugar) once it is eaten. When you know how much carbohydrate is in a certain food and combine that with the GI, then you have the glycemic load (GL). That's what really counts. The absolute best source for knowing the GL for just about every carb you ever hope to eat can be found at www.Mendosa.com. Don't be confused by the terms. **Glycemic index refers to the food. Glycemic load refers to the impact on your blood sugar level.**

Blood Sugar Response to the Glycemic Load

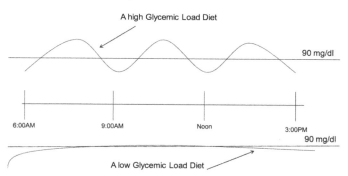

The graphic on page 113 represents how both high and low glycemic index foods can affect your blood sugar during a day. The upper line shows what happens if you eat simple carbs throughout the day. If you had a bagel (refined grain) and a donut with a cup of coffee for breakfast at around 6:00 am, by 9:00 am (or earlier), your blood sugar level would be below what is your normal steady state blood sugar level (represented by the 90 mg/dl line). Foods that are high on the glycemic index, such as a bagel, force the body to pump insulin into the blood to counter the rapid rise in blood sugar.

Unlike fighter pilots that learn to "lead the target" when gunning an aerial opponent, this insulin injection is in a tail chase and eventually ends up being more than needed to counter the rapid rise in the blood sugar level. Within an hour or two, the insulin overcompensates for the rise in blood sugar and actually lowers it below your normal, steady state blood sugar level (again, as represented by the 90 mg/dl line on the chart). Ninety milligrams (90 mg) per deciliter is used as a reference line and is considered a good blood glucose level. Your doctor will likely test "fasting glucose" and look for a reading below 100-110 mg/dl. Anything over 125 mg/dl is considered diabetic.

When blood sugar is low, we feel tired and often eat something to perk us up. Many of us have learned to select foods that rapidly pull us out of this low blood sugar (tired) state caused by too much insulin. The foods we choose are usually available in the break rooms of a typical office complex or at *7-Eleven*-type convenience stores. Unfortunately, these foods have both a high glycemic index and high calorie density. They include potato chips, cookies and other Red Light snack foods. I see this every day at work, where people are trying to manage their energy levels by routinely consuming high glycemic index foods. Is this what you're doing?

> When blood sugar is low, we feel tired and often eat something to perk us up.

Many of us manage our energy levels with calorie laden and high glycemic index foods causing our blood sugar levels to roller coaster throughout the day (as represented by the wavy line). If you've been doing this for years, you've more than likely found yourself stuck in this hellish cycle. We've learned to use quick-energy foods to manage our energy levels, but these foods deliver far more calories than can be burned each day. The result is weight gain and the loss of vitality and energy. Once we are overweight, our bodies are stressed energy-wise even to work in our mostly sedentary environments.

In the most severe cases, this high glycemic roller coaster is the only short-lived escape we have from that constant feeling of tiredness. I saw this happening with my sister in the years immediately prior to her death. Many of us choose foods throughout the day from vending machines and convenience stores that provide the absolute opposite of what our bodies need. These processed, high GI, calorie-dense, long shelf life foods are always available because they are logistically viable and deliver the most profit. The fresh foods you should be eating never seem to be available. It's no wonder that Americans are in such poor physical shape!

One of the most popular products these days is a 2-ounce drink called *5-Hour Energy*. According to the advertising, *5-Hour Energy* is specifically designed to perk you up mid-afternoon. What most people don't know is that this product contains up to 8,000 percent of the recommended daily value (DV) of vitamin B-12 and potentially dangerous levels of other B vitamins and folic acid. It is popular only because so many people don't eat correctly and their blood sugar has plummeted after that high glycemic load meal they had at lunchtime. If you eat right, you won't need the oral equivalent of a vitamin B injection after lunch each day.

If you wake up in the morning and eat a healthy and appropriately portioned breakfast of fruit, dairy, protein and whole grains with a low glycemic load, you'll find you don't get tired by mid-morning. This is due to your body slowly trickling insulin into your blood stream throughout the morning, which is represented by the slightly curved line on the bottom of the graph (Low Glycemic Load Diet).

With a slow trickle of insulin throughout the morning, your energy level remains relatively constant, and you'll find yourself eating in response to true hunger at lunchtime. If lunch is a combination of lean protein and complex carbohydrates (think low sodium turkey sandwich on whole wheat bread), along with veggies, fruits, and a dairy product, you'll again find yourself with plenty of energy until dinnertime.

I believe many Americans are overweight because they consume too many calories throughout the day in an attempt to manage their energy levels with high glycemic index foods. The unfortunate fact is that most of the prepared foods readily available to Americans, especially those who work away from their homes, are both calorie-dense and have a high glycemic index.

Although the good carbs vs. bad carbs information in advertisements is on the right track, it just doesn't tell the whole story. Low "glycemic index" foods are not the key to miracle weight loss as some of the plans want you to believe. The truth is that a daily diet that manages carbohydrate intake and portion control ("How Much") and includes other healthy Green Light foods, is how we should <u>all</u> eat. It's not just for those of us who are trying to lose weight or are diabetic. It's the way we were all designed to eat in the first place.

Many of the high glycemic index foods that adversely affect

your blood sugar were simply not available for most of humans' existence. That's why your body reacts negatively to them and is why you shouldn't eat them! If you're a diabetic, your doctor has prescribed a diet that helps control carbohydrate intake because your body is impaired in its ability to manage high glycemic index foods.

In order to lose weight, <u>you must reduce the calories you consume</u>. Simply changing the ratio of good and bad carbs (and even protein or fat) won't make you magically lose weight. Eating the right types of foods so that you're not managing your energy and blood sugar level with dense calories can accelerate your weight loss because you're consuming fewer calories. That's what really helps!

> Simply changing the ratio of good and bad carbs (and even protein or fat) won't make you magically lose weight.

The bottom line is that we should consciously choose the foods we eat, and in most cases, prepare it ourselves so we know what our meals contain. I achieved positive results in my weight loss journey because, as a "What" eater, I controlled most of the foods I ate. Don't let the local convenience store or office vending machine decide what you'll have for lunch. Too many of us eat foods with little thought of how they are affecting our overall health and waistline.

Study the Food Stoplight Charts. Virtually all of the Green Light foods, when eaten in appropriate portions, will help you manage your blood sugar. Notice that fruits, vegetables, proteins, dairy and grains are all represented. Truth be told, most healthy people who have achieved an appropriate weight for their height eat from all three of the Stoplight categories (green, yellow, red). It's how often and how much Yellow and Red Light foods they eat that makes the difference.

Yes, I'll have a Yellow Light food occasionally, and even Red Light food every once in a while. The important thing is how you define "occasionally" and "every once in a while." The fact remains that Green Light foods are the major part of my diet. You'll know you're doing it right if your weight is appropriate for your height and your blood pressure, blood sugar and lipid profile are all in the normal range. The metrics, or measurements, tell the truth.

If you routinely eat high glycemic index foods you're putting your long-term health at risk. These foods aren't what you were designed to eat and they'll tax your body's ability to function normally. On the other hand, there are many benefits from eating low glycemic index foods. They will help you:

- Lose weight, since you'll feel fuller for a longer time between meals
- Reduce your risk of heart disease
- Lower your bad cholesterol and raise your good cholesterol
- Have more energy
- Reduce your risk of diabetes
- Control your diabetes if you're already diabetic

Best Low-Glycemic Index (GI) Foods

You don't have to count calories to switch to healthier low GI foods. Instead, eat:

- Breakfast cereals with oats, barley and bran
- 100% whole wheat and other whole grain breads
- Basmati or doongara rice
- Fresh (or frozen) fruits and vegetables
- Whole wheat pasta and quinoa
- Lots of salad vegetables with a low-oil based dressing or salsa.

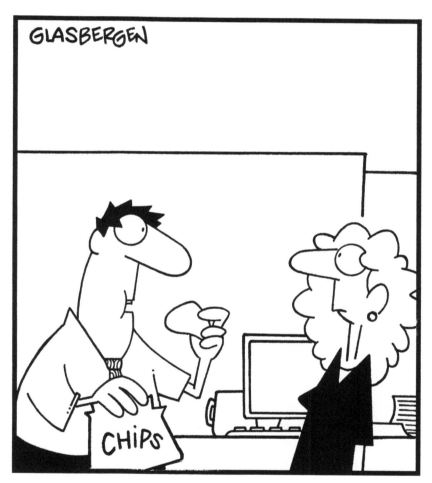

"They tried adding healthy snacks to the office vending machines, but all that rotting fruit made the candy bars taste bad."

22

Antioxidants and Supplements

Antioxidants

> Antioxidants are natural compounds found in many foods that _may_ lower the risk of cancer, help reduce heart disease, lower blood pressure and purportedly, slow the effects of aging.

Well into my weight loss journey I heard about something called antioxidants and free radicals. Being in the intelligence field at the time, I was relieved to find out that antioxidants are not nasty chemical weapons used by some terrorist organization called the Free Radicals. What I did find out was that there is much misinformation out there concerning antioxidants, mostly due to food manufacturing labels and advertisements.

I learned that antioxidants are natural compounds found in many foods that _may_ lower the risk of cancer, help reduce heart disease, lower blood pressure and purportedly, slow the effects of aging. When we say antioxidants, what we generally mean is vitamins E and C. It's important to have both in your diet since vitamin E is the most abundant fat-soluble antioxidant in the body, while vitamin C is the most abundant water-soluble antioxidant. Water-based vitamin C _may_ help you fight off the effects of pollution and second-hand smoke. Fat-soluble vitamin E _could_ be your protection against cardiovascular disease and the formation of plaque in your arteries. Both come into play when dealing with free radicals.

To understand free radicals, it may help to borrow your tenth grader's chemistry book (which I needed) to review the basics of atoms. They have a nucleus and contain neutrons, protons and electrons. Normally, electrons are paired in an outer shell, often by sharing electrons as part of the chemical bonding process. Most of the time the chemical bonds don't break in a way that leave an unpaired electron, but when they do, a free radical is formed. These free radicals will attack stable molecules in the hunt for the missing electron. Here's where antioxidants come into play. This hunt for a free electron will result in a chain reaction with other stable molecules unless antioxidants (vitamins E and C) are present.

The beauty of antioxidants is that they are stable with or without paired electrons. Lots of antioxidants result in stable electron-paired cells. The bottom line is that without sufficient antioxidants in your body, you could be setting yourself up for life-threatening diseases. Unfortunately, the research on how well antioxidants protect us against cancer and heart disease is all over the map, including the possibility that they may only help people with certain genetic characteristics.

You may recall I said that chances are you'll eventually die of heart-related disease or cancer unless you're one of the unlucky few who die in a traumatic accident. Achieving an appropriate weight for our height is one of the best things we can all do to delay the onset of heart disease and cancer, with the added benefit of improving our quality of life along the way.

Antioxidants may be a critical part of both the weight-loss process and disease prevention, not as much due to the benefit of the antioxidants (we're still learning what they are), but because of the foods that contain them. In other words, if you eat healthy foods for weight loss and good health, you're most likely eating foods with lots of antioxidants. Translation: If you eat healthy foods, you don't need to be too concerned about antioxidants. That being said, I've included a short list of my favorite antioxidant-rich foods below so you'd know what types of foods I'm discussing.

> If you eat healthy foods, you don't need to be too concerned about antioxidants.

This list is a great place to start getting your five to eight servings of antioxidant-rich foods each day.

Ed's List of Best Antioxidant-Rich Foods:

Beans (e.g., red, black, kidney, pinto)

Berries (e.g., blueberries, raspberries, cranberries, strawberries)

Apples (e.g., Red Delicious, Granny Smith, Gala)

Raisins, plums, prunes, sweet cherries, red grapes, oranges, grapefruit, kiwi, pomegranate, pineapple)

Nuts (e.g., pecans, walnuts, almonds, hazelnuts)

Vegetables (e.g., artichokes, kale, spinach, broccoli, cauliflower, corn, tomatoes, potatoes, carrots, eggplant, mini-peppers, red, green and yellow bell peppers, onions, garlic, chili peppers, Brussels and alfalfa sprouts)

Whole grains and cereals (e.g., barley, oats, corn, millet)

Tea, pomegranate juice, red wine

You may see some foods (and liquid supplements) that list the "oxygen radical absorbance capacity" or ORAC value. Generally, if a product has to tout its ORAC value it is probably a marketing scam. You'll never see a pint of blueberries touting its ORAC value, and trust me, they're loaded with antioxidants.

Another thing, don't fall for those high-priced juice scams, most notably *Mangosteen* supplements and *Gogi* berry-based juices or powder. If you want to spend $30 on 25 ounces of juice, I suggest that you look to the legitimate wine merchants of the world. You'll get plenty of antioxidants, a fantastic bottle of wine (probably two or three), and won't feel "amazingly stupid" (to quote an internet blogger) for wasting your money on these juice scams. If you're a teetotaler, I suggest *Langers All Pomegranate* juice (my favorite). You'll get two quarts of pure pomegranate juice for about seven dollars with all the antioxidant benefits and still have 23 bucks left in your pocket.

Don't be like many of the people I see that use overpriced antioxidant products (*Noni*, *Mangosteen* and *Acai* tablets and juices) as a way to feel good about taking ownership of their health. What they are really doing is outsourcing their health (and sometimes weight loss) to these heavily marketed products that have never been proven in real studies to do anything other than lighten their wallet.

Unless you're willing to eat right and exercise, you're only fooling yourself if you think you can positively affect / improve your health with these high-priced, useless products. Again, stick with healthy foods and don't worry about things like ORAC value.

> Stick with healthy foods and don't worry about things like ORAC value.

Yet another outrageous claim is that you can lose weight while eating antioxidant-rich dark chocolate. Oh, if it only could be true! Yes, dark chocolate (not milk chocolate) has various health benefits, but the reality is that it's a fairly high-calorie food that contains saturated fat, even if it is made with "unprocessed cocoa" as claimed by the makers of *Xocai*. I definitely enjoy dark chocolate (a *superfood*), but I would never eat three pieces a day to try to lose weight or pay more than a dollar for a 12-gram piece of chocolate.

A 2010 German study linked the consumption of dark chocolate with lower blood pressure and a reduction in cardiovascular disease. The study participants consumed just six grams (30 calories) of dark chocolate (about one and a half *Hershey's Kisses*) per day. Their blood pressure went down by an average of three points systolic (top number), and two points diastolic (bottom number). The researchers noted that

Bottom line: Eat healthy Green Light foods, exercise, and be wary of any product that has to tout its antioxidant benefits or ORAC values.

it doesn't help to eat more chocolate because the added calories start to outweigh the benefits of the flavonoids* in the dark chocolate. The distinguished Dr. Lawrence Appel of the John Hopkins School of Medicine commented on the study and gives us some great advice. He said that while eating six grams of dark chocolate wouldn't hurt, the best way to lower your blood pressure is to "Lose weight and consume less salt."

Bottom line: Eat healthy Green Light foods, exercise, and be wary of any product that has to tout its antioxidant benefits or ORAC values.

Supplements

In my mind, there are only three supplements worth considering and another one that demonstrates the success of supplement marketing. In relative order of their importance to your good health, they are:

Vitamin D

Recent studies have identified the lack of vitamin D as a causal factor in several types of cancers. Many Americans may have insufficient levels of vitamin D in their blood due to their diet and lifestyle. Since the sun is a natural source of vitamin D, contributing factors for our low vitamin D levels may include living in the northern regions of the United States and our increased use of high SPF sunscreen. Cancer rates increase among the general population the further north you live in the United States, and some researchers believe the connection is the lower blood levels of vitamin D.

History tells us that when our ancestors moved to northern latitudes, their skin turned lighter because nature favored fair-

---

*Flavonoids are brightly colored plant pigments that occur naturally in most fresh fruits and vegetables. Many of these compounds serve as antioxidants or contribute in other ways to maintain health. (Source: GreenFacts)

skinned humans' ability to absorb vitamin D from the sun. Without sufficient vitamin D, humans can develop rickets, a bone weakening disease that was prevalent in the US until the 1950s. Natural selection favored the ability to absorb vitamin D since a woman with a weakened pelvis (due to rickets) couldn't support the rigors of child bearing.

Our Alaskan brethren are the only northern dwelling people that have retained their dark skin because they get all the vitamin D they need from the fish they eat. So we can follow their lead and eat plenty of vitamin D-rich fish, take a vitamin D supplement (D_3 is best) or both. Check with your doctor or nutritionist before taking any supplement, even a daily multi-vitamin if you take any medication.

Fast-forward to today when most of us have a diet that doesn't contain much vitamin D in spite of all the vitamin D-fortified foods available (milk, yogurt, cereals, etc). Without many chances for absorbing vitamin D from the sun during a typical work week, the only way to ensure that we get enough vitamin D is to choose the right foods and take a vitamin D supplement.

> Check with your doctor or nutritionist before taking any supplement, even a daily multi-vitamin if you take any medication.

Vitamin D-rich foods include salmon, catfish (but eating it fried kills any health benefit), shrimp and tuna, as well as fortified foods such as milk, yogurt, soymilk, oatmeal and many breakfast cereals. In addition, most multi-vitamins contain 400 International Units (IU) of vitamin D. You need at least 1,000 IUs a day, so vitamin D-rich foods need to be part of your overall plan even if you take a multi-vitamin.

For some people, it may be best to just take 800 - 1,000 (IUs) of vitamin D_3 each day as a supplement. This is especially true for the elderly, those with poor diets, dark skinned individuals and those of us who live north of 40 degrees latitude here in the

United States. That's north of Denver and Philadelphia. There's just not enough sunlight in the northern regions in winter to naturally get the amount of vitamin D you need.

Although I am relatively fair skinned and use sunscreen when outdoors for a significant amount of time, I'll spend about 10 minutes out in the sun during the summertime wearing just shorts and a t-shirt. Doing this a couple times a week can provide you with all the vitamin D you need. For comparison, a day at the beach with unprotected skin (not advised) can provide the equivalent of 25,000 IUs of vitamin D.

The takeaway here is that you just need a little natural sun and a fairly good diet to keep your level of vitamin D in the right range during the summer. During the winter, most of us should take a vitamin D_3 supplement, especially those of us that live in the northern half of the US.

Post-menopausal women should consider taking a vitamin D supplement all year long due to the fact that nearly a third of the women studied had vitamin D levels below the normal range. This also helps in the fight against osteoporosis, but a vitamin D supplement has to be combined with dietary (not supplement) calcium to be truly effective. Calcium-rich foods include milk, yogurt, cottage cheese, broccoli, kale, green beans, almonds, walnuts, red kidney beans, chick peas (as in hummus), apricots, figs, oranges and even salmon. We keep coming back to the same theme—eating right is critical to good health!

> During the winter, most of us should take a vitamin D_3 supplement, especially those of us that live in the northern half of the US.

It appears that individuals who suffer from osteoarthritis can also benefit from a vitamin D supplement. I had my vitamin D level checked before I considered taking vitamin D for my arthritis, and even without supplements I was in the normal range, mostly due to the fact that I love and eat a great deal of fish. If you don't like fish, have your vitamin D level checked and also consider taking an omega-3 supplement (discussed below). This can get very confusing; therefore you really need to discuss your supplement strategy with your doctor who can advise you relative to your current medications.

> Many of us could benefit from more omega-3 in our diet.

Omega-3

Even with a nearly perfect diet, which few of us have, it appears that many of us could benefit from more omega-3 in our diet. Omega-3 can get a bit confusing since it comes from two different sources. One type, alpha-linolenic acid (ALA), comes from flax, walnuts and dark green leafy vegetables. The second, eicosapentaenoic acid (EPA) and docosahexaenoic Acid (DHA), comes from fish. Technically, the body can convert the ALA fats into the more desirable EPA and DHA, but today's high levels of omega-6 in the typical American's diet all but shut this process down.

Therefore, if you don't like fish, you're more likely to be deficient in those EPA and DHA essential fatty acids that your body cannot produce on its own. Several studies not only support the effectiveness of omega-3 supplements, but also indicate that omega-3s may help achieve and maintain good cholesterol levels, improve cognitive function, decrease abnormal heart rhythms and help prevent stroke and cancer. The only solution if you don't like or can't eat fish is to take an omega-3 EPA and DHA supplement.

> A quality multi-vitamin is a good idea for most Americans since our diets are often deficient in one or more essential nutrients.

Multi-Vitamins

Once again, Mom was right. We should take our vitamins. A quality multi-vitamin is a good idea for most Americans since our diets are often deficient in one or more essential nutrients.

That being said, some recent studies suggest that too much folic acid may raise the risk of colon cancer and too much selenium could be linked to diabetes.

Those of us with nutrient-rich diets might want to take a multi-vitamin just every other day. My doctor not only approves this approach, but likes the numbers he sees on the results of my annual physical blood test. I can't say enough about how important it is to inform your doctor about any supplements you take, even a multi-vitamin or an aspirin.

Supplement Marketing Success: Glucosamine and Chondroitin.

I have included glucosamine and chondroitin only because I know so many people who take them, although I must admit up front that there's little scientific or research evidence to support their use. Here's what we do know: Glucosamine is an amino sugar found in cartilage and other connective tissue, while chondroitin sulfate is a complex carbohydrate that may help cartilage retain water.

Since I have moderate osteoarthritis, I've discussed the use of glucosamine and chondroitin with my rheumatologist, a very talented doctor at the National Naval Medical Center (Bethesda). He echoes what all the studies have concluded, that there is no compelling, positive evidence for using glucosamine and chondroitin. He told me what he tells all his patients, "Go ahead and take them if they make you feel better, because they won't hurt you if they don't."

One of the best (and my favorite) study about the effectiveness of these supplements was conducted by the National Institutes of Health (NIH). One reason I like the "Glucosamine/Chondroitin Arthritis Intervention Trial (GAIT)" study is that it wasn't funded by the makers of glucosamine and chondroitin. You wouldn't believe how many studies are funded by companies so they can use the results to market their product.

These companies know that most people will never read the studies, but will hear the 30-second news report that's says, "Dark chocolate lowers blood pressure." We now know the truth about that study. Of course, you never hear about the company-funded studies that bomb and are never published (like the ones that try to prove that diet soda helps you lose weight).

The GAIT study was conducted double-blind, meaning both the patients and doctors were unaware who was getting the supplements and who was getting the placebos. They also included celecoxib (*Celebrex*), a non-steroidal anti-inflammatory pain drug, and compared it to a placebo to validate the study design. GAIT has all the elements of a good study, especially to a study junkie like me.

The results, while a little difficult to digest, are taken directly from the Backgrounder portion of the study at the NIH web-site (http://nccam.nih.gov/research/results/gait/qa.htm). The study found:

- "Participants taking the positive control, celecoxib, experienced statistically significant pain relief versus taking the placebo—about 70 percent of those taking celecoxib had a 20 percent or greater reduction in pain versus about 60 percent for the placebo."

- "Overall, there were no significant differences between the other treatments tested (glucosamine and chondroitin) and the placebo."

What this tells us is that a known pain reliever (*Celebrex*) not only proved it works, but also validated a study that found no significant pain relief between the glucosamine and chondroitin and a sugar pill (placebo).

The study did go on to explain that a very small subset of test participants with what is defined as "moderate-to-severe (arthritis) pain," did see statistical pain relief (79 percent) when

> Unlike glucosamine and chondroitin, many supplements are dangerous for people with certain medical conditions when taken in too high of doses and when combined with certain prescription medications.

compared to those that took the placebo (54 percent), but the numbers were too small to draw any positive conclusions.

What amazes me is that 60 percent of the placebo takers in the *Celebrex* portion of the study and 54 percent of the placebo takers in the glucosamine and chondroitin study group saw the same 20 percent or greater reduction in pain. How is it possible that such a large portion of the study participants reported statistically significant pain relief when they were just taking a sugar pill?

I believe this study demonstrates that there is a powerful "psychological" effect when it comes to taking supplements (and proven pain relievers). If a well-run, tightly controlled study like GAIT can have more than half the placebo takers claim statistically significant pain relief, we can see why the marketing efforts of every possible supplement under the sun have been so successful.

The companies that sell supplements have seen the results of these studies and don't have to employ too many Harvard Business School grads to figure out that there's a very lucrative market for supplement sales. If just taking a sugar pill makes people feel better, why not a bottle of pills at 20 bucks a pop? Unfortunately, unlike glucosamine and chondroitin, many supplements are dangerous for people with certain medical conditions when taken in too high of doses and when combined with certain prescription medications.

The Government Accountability Office (GAO) published a report (GAO-10-662T) in May 2010 that highlighted some of the deceptive and questionable marketing practices as well as the potentially dangerous advice they received from (mostly) supplement retailers and marketers. The GAO found that many online retailers were guilty of claiming that certain supplements were effective in treating or curing serious conditions such as diabetes, cancer and cardiovascular disease.

The GAO also reported **dangerous advice** from supplement marketers, such as stating that ginkgo biloba can be safely taken with aspirin, which in fact, is unsafe because it can increase the risk of bleeding. The same GAO report "found trace amounts of at least one potentially hazardous contaminant in 37 of 40 herbal dietary supplement products tested." While none were "considered to pose an acute toxicity hazard" the GAO found lead, mercury, cadmium, arsenic and residues from pesticides. When supplements are taken every day, or in large doses, these "trace" amounts of contaminants (especially lead) can build up in our blood stream and negatively affect our overall health.

All of this information emphasizes the fact that we need to be particularly mindful of what supplements we take, which ones we give our children, and from what source we buy our supplements. My advice is to approach all supplements cautiously, limit the amounts you take, read the labels closely and ensure they are manufactured by well-known and respected companies. Most importantly, as I have indicated throughout this chapter, don't take any drug or supplement without your doctor's okay

Bottom Line:

More is not necessarily better when it comes to supplements and vitamins. It can be dangerous if you take high doses of any vitamin in supplement form. Toxicity ranges vary widely from more than a little is too much (vitamin E) all the way to you're probably not getting enough (vitamin D). Additionally, the value of antioxidants may be more than just the vitamins we have identified. Researchers have identified so many compounds in antioxidant

> More is not necessarily better when it comes to supplements and vitamins. It can be dangerous if you take high doses of any vitamin in supplement form.

rich foods the only way we can be sure we are getting the benefit is to eat the foods nature has provided.

Many people mistakenly think they can take a pill to make up for a nutrient-poor diet. While a multi-vitamin is a good idea as discussed previously, what the supplement companies won't tell you is that there are some nutrients (potassium, magnesium, calcium) that are not easily replaced in a poor diet in supplement form. If you really want to improve your health, eat healthy Green Light foods, exercise and leave most of the mega-marketed supplements on the store shelf.

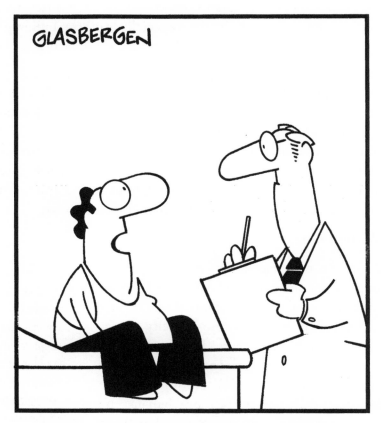

"Eat less and exercise more? That's the most ridiculous fad diet I've heard of yet!"

23

Label Reading 101

By now you have learned a great deal about the weight-loss process and know how to manage your overall good health. Yet there is still at least one critical skill you need: label reading. First, let's acknowledge that there are legions of very bright, well-educated Madison Avenue marketers that make lots of money by figuring out how to sell us new products. The energy drink craze, primarily marketed to our teenagers and young adults, is a great example. In a twist on the tag line from the movie "Field of Dreams," they know that if they market it, we—especially the youth—will come and buy it.

McDonald's "Super Size" meal plan* was one of the most successful food marketing campaigns in American history. It was an absolutely brilliant idea. I remember that when I frequented fast food establishments, I felt stupid if I didn't get the super size order. For just a few extra dimes (back then) I'd get considerably more soft drink and fries. At that time, I didn't realize that I was adding significantly both to the restaurant's profits and to my own rapidly expanding waistline.

The marketing folks figured out that it only cost pennies to give us the extra product since the smaller sized items already paid for the food container, building, equipment, insurance, and transportation and labor costs. This is one example of how they understood human behavior extremely well and how we unconsciously played right into their hands. Food manufacturers try to influence us in the same way with every box, container or package of food or drink we buy in this country. It's important to understand what we're really getting when we purchase any food or beverage.

*Prior to the 2004 release of the Movie *"Super Size Me"*, McDonald's announced that it would stop selling supersized drinks and fries.

I found I really had to study food labeling and packaging to understand them. I also discovered that it was useful to know what was required by law, what food manufacturers can claim on their packaging, and how important it is to bring your glasses to the grocery store.

As far as labeling is concerned, there are three things to look for. First is the large lettering on the packaging that tells you what the Madison Avenue folks wants you to know. If you just read the package label, you're not getting all the facts. Remember, it was the Madison Avenue types that came up with the idea to splash "zero trans fat" on products that never had any trans fat in the first place, and "zero carbs" on products that were loaded with salt and fat. Second, look to the ingredient list to find out what the food product really contains. This is invariably in very small print and why you need your glasses.

Finally, refer to the Nutrition Facts Label (required by law), to see how many calories and how much fat, sodium, fiber and added sugar the product contains. It's also important to note the number of servings because oftentimes a packaged product like chicken pot pie will indicate it contains two servings, meaning you need to double the calories, sodium and fat if you plan on consuming the entire pie yourself (and who wouldn't?).

Here's what else I learned:

Most of the information on food packaging labels falls into a category defined as "structure and function claims." The Food and Drug Administration (FDA) allows structure and function claims to *"describe the role of a nutrient or dietary ingredient intended to affect normal structure or function in humans."*

A good example of this is "calcium builds strong bones." This can be printed on a product label even if the amount of calcium in the product wouldn't positively affect your bones unless you consumed 20 regular servings. So while the product does have calcium and "normally" calcium does in fact help build strong bones, this particular product may or may not actually help your bones grow stronger. It's up to you to know how much calcium the product is providing in relation to what your body needs each day to actually influence strong bones. Hang on, it gets worse!

Manufacturers can also make "health claims" and "nutrient content" claims on food labels. Health claims describe the relationship between a food or ingredient, and its *ability in reducing risk of disease or health-related conditions.*" A good example is the apparently true health claim on *Cheerios* that states "Clinically Proven to Help Lower Cholesterol." This is the only type of claim that gets FDA scrutiny. Manufacturers must petition the FDA to review prevailing scientific literature and studies to ensure the claim meets a *"Significant scientific agreement standard to determine that the nutrient/disease relationship is well established."*

Even with the requirement for scientific agreement, the FDA has recently allowed *Fritos* corn chips to be described as "supporting a healthy heart." This is apparently due to the fact that *Frito-Lay*, a subsidiary of *Pepsi* (annual sales of nearly 45 billion dollars) has the clout to convince the FDA that by replacing saturated fat with sunflower oil (yes, an omega-6 fat we get way too much of already), *Fritos* are now a healthy, wholesome food. This is what you're up against with product labeling in this country.

Nutrient claims "characterize the level of a nutrient in a food" using terms such as free, high, low, more, reduced and light (lite). Look in your pantry to see how many food products have these claims. Examples include "reduced sodium (90 mg)" since that could be considered good when compared to the daily maximum of 2,400 mg.

Always check the serving size to ensure that you're only eating a single serving containing just the 90 mg stated. Some manufacturers make serving sizes so small that you might be getting two to three times that amount in what you'd consider a normal serving. Another example is "reduced fat" which means it has 25 percent less fat than the full fat version of the product. Be careful though. Even 25 percent less fat could be serving up a tremendous amount of total fat and calories in a normal serving.

For what it's worth, neither structure and function claims or nutrient claims receive the same oversight as health claims, and must only be *"Truthful and not misleading."* Walking that thin *"Truthful and not misleading"* line is an art form and is why Madison Avenue advertisers get the big bucks.

For example, let's take a look at a very popular processed food (*Cheerios*) and see what information the packaging label, ingredients list and Nutrition Fact Label tell us. *Cheerios* is touting that it is a whole grain food (in two places) and part of a heart healthy diet. It also contains a Health Claim, stating *Cheerios* may reduce the risk of heart disease. I checked, and that is, in fact, backed up with study evidence on whole grain oats. A quick glance at the ingredients list confirms that "Whole Grain Oats" is the first ingredient, followed by the modified corn starch, sugar and salt that is in virtually all processed foods. *Cheerios* also contains many of the vitamins that your body needs and can be hard to get*.

We're not done yet. The Nutrition Facts Label confirms that, all-in-all, this probably isn't a bad food choice, as processed foods go. Note that a one cup serving is only 100 calories, but delivers three grams of fiber and protein, without an excess of sugars (only one gram) and sodium (160 mg). Fat is a reasonable two grams with half the poly and monounsaturated fats that are in the better category as far as fat is concerned.

Finally, *Cheerios* is a good source of potassium as well as a

---

* MultiGrain Cheerios have the same 3 grams of fiber as regular Cheerios, but come with six times the added sugar for the same size serving.

*host of other required nutrients with fairly healthy percent Daily Values (DV) of everything from vitamin A to Zinc. Also note that a single cup of *Cheerios* provides 50 percent of the recommended DV of folic acid (vitamin B_9).

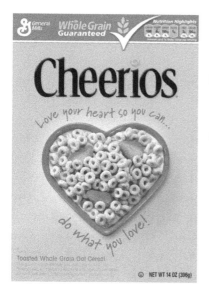

Nutrition Facts

Serving Size 1 cup (28g)
   Children Under 4 - 3/4 cup (21g)
Servings Per Container about 14
   Children Under 4 - about 19

Amount Per Serving	Cheerios	with 1/2 cup skim milk	Cereal for Children Under 4
Calories	100	140	80
Calories from Fat	15	20	10
		% Daily Value	
Total Fat 2g*	**3%**	**3%**	1.5g
Saturated Fat 0g	**0%**	**3%**	0g
Trans Fat 0g			0g
Polyunsaturated Fat 0.5g			0g
Monounsaturated Fat 0.5g			0g
Cholesterol 0mg	**0%**	**1%**	0mg
Sodium 160mg	**7%**	**9%**	120mg
Potassium 170mg	**5%**	**11%**	130mg
Total Carbohydrate 20g	**7%**	**9%**	15g
Dietary Fiber 3g	**11%**	**11%**	2g
Soluble Fiber 1g			0g
Sugars 1g			1g
Other Carbohydrate 17g			12g
Protein 3g			2g

		% Daily Value	
Protein	-	-	9%
Vitamin A	10%	15%	10%
Vitamin C	10%	10%	10%
Calcium	10%	25%	8%
Iron	45%	45%	50%
Vitamin D	10%	25%	6%
Thiamin	25%	30%	35%
Riboflavin	25%	35%	35%
Niacin	25%	25%	35%
Vitamin B_6	25%	25%	45%
Folic Acid	50%	50%	60%
Vitamin B_{12}	25%	35%	30%
Phosphorus	10%	25%	8%
Magnesium	10%	10%	10%
Zinc	25%	30%	30%

* Amount in cereal. A serving of cereal plus skim milk provides 2g total fat (0.5g saturated fat, 1g monounsaturated fat), less than 5mg cholesterol, 220mg sodium, 380mg potassium, 26g total carbohydrate (7g sugars) and 8g protein.
** Percent Daily Values are based on a 2,000 calorie diet. Your daily values may be higher or lower depending on your calorie needs.

	Calories	2,000	2,500
Total Fat	Less than	65g	80g
Sat Fat	Less than	20g	25g
Cholesterol	Less than	300mg	300mg
Sodium	Less than	2,400mg	2,400mg
Potassium		3,500mg	3,500mg
Total Carbohydrate		300g	375g
Dietary Fiber		25g	30g
Protein		50g	65g

Ingredients: Whole Grain Oats (includes the oat bran), **Modified Corn Starch, Sugar, Salt, Tripotassium Phosphate, Oat Fiber, Wheat Starch. Vitamin E** (mixed tocopherols) **Added to Preserve Freshness.**

Vitamins and Minerals:
Calcium Carbonate, Iron and Zinc (mineral nutrients), **Vitamin C** (sodium ascorbate), **A B Vitamin** (niacinamide), **Vitamin B_6** (pyridoxine hydrochloride), **Vitamin A** (palmitate), **Vitamin B_2** (riboflavin), **Vitamin B_1** (thiamin mononitrate), **A B Vitamin** (folic acid), **Vitamin B_{12}, Vitamin D_3**.

You'll recall that too much folic acid in the diet (from both foods and supplements) has been linked to an increase in colon cancer. So if you have a nutrient rich diet (with all those Green Light foods you're eating now) and eat fortified breakfast cereals, you need to be careful about the supplements you take, even a daily multi-vitamin. That's why many doctors recommend a multi-vitamin every other day for those of us that really take this nutrition stuff seriously.

Typical Label Claims

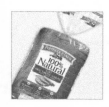

"100% natural"

Even Pepperidge Farm, manufacturer of some of the healthiest bread, can't help splashing "100% natural" on the label. Do you know what 100% natural means? Don't feel bad, neither does the FDA. In fact, the FDA, after being petitioned for a definition by both the *Sugar Association Trade Group* and *Sara Lee*, decided that *"natural will remain undefined."* The FDA website says *"we're not sure how high of an issue it is for consumers."* Additionally, the FDA sited *"resource limitations and other agency priorities,"* which I don't doubt. As I've stated previously, here is a sterling example of how "you are on your own."

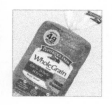

"100 % whole wheat"

It should be easy to understand whether or not a food is made with whole wheat or other healthy whole grains. But it's really confusing. Now that our food manufacturers know we're interested in eating complex carbohydrates (whole grains), they have complicated it to the point that we really have to know how to read and understand their packaging label, the Nutrition Facts Label and the ingredients list to know what we are eating.

Here's what you should do: When buying bread, rolls, English muffins, etc, look for "100% whole wheat" on the label and then check the list of ingredients just to be sure. Many manufacturers will splash terms on their labels that say "Whole Grain," "Whole Grain Blend" or "Harvest Wheat" while using mostly refined white, durum and rice flour to supplement a small portion of the whole wheat grain. It's complicated because we want our bread to be "100% whole wheat," which is one of the many whole grains, but if the label says "whole grain" it probably has only a small portion of "whole wheat." Let me explain.

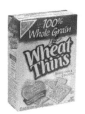

"Whole Grain"

Whole grains are any of the cereal grains that contain bran and germ as well as the endosperm. For comparison, refined grain products contain only the endosperm. Whole grains include wheat, oats, barley, brown rice, corn, quinoa and rye. If bread is baked using only a portion of one of these whole grains, the FDA allows the label to state "whole grain." It is then up to the consumer to check the ingredients list to figure out how much of the whole grain comes into play.

If a whole grain is the first ingredient listed, it's probably OK since manufacturers must list the predominant ingredient first, followed by the others in decreasing order. If the ingredients list doesn't mention the whole grain until third or fourth, then the bread is more than likely made with <u>mostly</u> refined grain. Remember, it's the 100 percent whole grains (in bread it's mostly 100 percent whole wheat) that makes you feel full (satiated) and provides the most health benefit.

> If a whole grain is the first ingredient listed, it's probably OK since manufacturers must list the predominant ingredient first, followed by the others in decreasing order.

Breads that have mostly refined grains have a high glycemic index and have a negative impact on your blood sugar as discussed in Chapter 21. Bread products can only state "100% whole wheat" if they are in fact made with <u>only</u> whole wheat.

Another bread labeling trick is to list "wheat flour" or even the trickier "100% wheat flour" as the first ingredient, leading some to think the bread is made with whole wheat. Many of these breads are even baked to look like whole wheat bread, but contain mostly refined grains. "Wheat flour" by FDA definition is refined grain. Some bread products will list whole grains (wheat, barley, oats) as the second and third ingredients, which means they do have some whole grains, but are still mostly refined grains (first ingredient) and not good for you.

On the other hand, many store-bought pizza crusts list "whole wheat flour" as the first ingredient, and are in fact, made with whole grain. It's possible to eat (somewhat) healthy "whole grain" bread that isn't 100% whole wheat as long as the first ingredient is a whole grain. If you are still confused, don't feel bad, many people have difficulty understanding this. My suggestion is to simply endeavor to buy bread that says it is "100% whole wheat" or that lists a whole grain as the first ingredient.

> My suggestion is to simply endeavor to buy bread that says it is "100% whole wheat" or that lists a whole grain as the first ingredient.

If you're not currently eating 100 percent whole wheat bread, give it a try and see if you don't really like the taste and feel better after eating it. In July 2010 the Nielsen Company reported that for the first time in US supermarket history, the 52-week total dollar sale of packaged "wheat" bread topped that of "white" bread. This indicates that Americans are finally eating more whole grains. Please note: Store bought pre-packaged rye and pumpernickel breads are mostly refined grains and not whole grain!

While our dizzying discussion of 100 percent whole wheat focused on whole grain bread, there are other whole grain products you'll probably be interested in eating. One is the aforementioned *Cheerios*, which states "Whole Grain Oat Cereal" on the label. The ingredients list shows "Whole Grain

Oats" as the first ingredient which is good, but then lists "Oat Bran" (fifth ingredient) and "Oat Fiber" (eighth) as additional ingredients. These fifth and eighth ingredients are not "whole grains," but again any product that lists a whole grain as its first ingredient is probably a good food choice.

"Multi-Grain"

Multi-Grain generally just means that a product has several different grains (wheat, barley, oats, etc.), probably even some whole grain, but you have to check the ingredients list to know for sure. Another claim is "8 or 12-Grain" but often the product doesn't contain much in the way of "whole grains" but is mostly several different refined grains that constitute the advertised eight or twelve grains.

Additionally, beware of claims that state, "provides 25% of your daily fiber" since many manufacturers are adding "isolated fibers" such as inulin, maltodextrin and polydextrose. Whatever they are, they don't provide the health benefit that 100% whole grain does.

"Good" or "Excellent Source of Whole Grains"

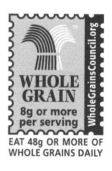

Be aware of terms like "Good" or "Excellent Source of Whole Grains" unless the product carries the "Whole Grains Council" stamp of approval. Due to typical FDA dithering on regulation of what exactly "Whole Grain" should mean, the food industry created the "Whole Grains Council" and came up with a stamp to help us find the healthy whole grains.

When you see the Whole Grain stamp, it means you're getting "at least half a serving (eight grams)" of whole grain ingredients. Before we get too excited about this stamp, I should tell you that I've seen it on products like *Multi-grain Cheese Puffs*. The goal, of course, is to eat your daily requirement of fiber and whole grains without excessive calories. The *Multi-grain Cheese Puffs* are probably not the smartest way to get your whole grains.

As I indicated earlier, choosing healthy (packaged) foods is a three-step process:

First check out the claims on the packaging, then see if the Nutrition Facts Label and the Ingredients List back up what the Madison Ave folks are trying to sell you. While a good portion of your food shouldn't even have a package (think fresh produce and other Green Light foods), with a little practice you'll be able to spot the best foods to feed your family.

One of the things that surprised me on the FDA web-site was that the FDA makes the assumption that consumers know to look at the first ingredient when evaluating a product's whole grain content. Good thing we know that now! If you really want to become an expert on reading the Nutrition Facts Label and a product's Ingredients List, visit the FDA web-site's "How to Understand and Use the Nutrition Facts Label." Find it at: http://www.fda.gov/food/labelingnutrition/consumer information/ucm078889.htm.

Other "Examples" of Food Product Labeling

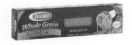 When you buy pasta products, understand that ingredients such as "Wheat flour," "Semolina" and "Durum wheat" generally mean that some part of the whole grain is missing. It's not "whole wheat." *Barilla*, maker of my favorite thin spaghetti, does a great job with their product marketing and packaging. Directly beneath their *Barilla* logo, they state "Whole Grain" and then, in print large enough to read without your glasses, they state that the spaghetti is "Made with 51% Whole Wheat." A check of the ingredients confirms this and lists, in order, "Whole Durum Wheat Flour", followed by "Semolina, Durum Wheat Flour (note it doesn't say "Whole") and "Oat Fiber."

This label makes it clear to me that I am getting 51 percent whole grain in my spaghetti, and that the rest of the grains are the semolina and durum flours that have part of the grain missing. This is okay, since many people, including my wife, find 100 percent whole wheat pasta a little too chewy. A serving of *Barilla* spaghetti delivers a solid six grams of dietary fiber (you should get 25-50 grams per day), just two grams of sugar, seven grams of protein, and zero milligrams of sodium (2,400 mg per day maximum). Choose the right spaghetti sauce, zest it up with onions, bell peppers and a little basil, and you have a delicious, low sodium, high fiber, healthy meal for your family. Healthy eating can be fun!

While the spaghetti label above notes the FDA's recommendation for fiber and sodium, it doesn't give us guidelines on sugar and protein other than advice to limit added sugars. Many healthy foods (fruit, vegetables, milk) contain naturally occurring sugars. It's the added ones we want to identify and limit, such as corn syrup, high-fructose corn syrup, fruit juice concentrate, maltose, dextrose, sucrose, honey, and maple syrup. Yogurt, a generally healthy food choice, can contain significant added sugar. Be sure to check the Nutrition Facts Label and Ingredients List.

My advice, especially for women, is to ensure you eat some protein at every meal. Men don't seem to have a problem with getting protein, probably because we eat too many hot dogs, hamburgers, chicken wings, etc. when watching sports. Not an entirely good thing, I admit!

Planters does a good job with package labeling, especially with its "Sensible Solutions" product line. Planters has a great natural product to begin with (nuts) and doesn't have to go far to make it healthy. The smoked almonds have half the sodium of its regular almonds and taste great, but still contain the fiber, protein, antioxidant vitamin E and the mostly poly and mono unsaturated fats you want. I eat some type of nut nearly every day, but just a handful, because they do have plenty of calories and (good) fat.

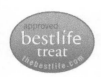

You may see a seal on some products for Bob Green's *Bestlife Program*. I trust this seal because Bob is not a food manufacturer. He only endorses products he feels meet the *Bestlife* lifestyle and I haven't seen it on any cheese puffs. Foods that carry the *Bestlife* seal include *Smart Balance, Lean Cuisine, Barilla Whole Grain Pasta, Bertolli Olive Oil, Lipton Teas, Florida Citrus, Yoplait Yogurt, Cheerios* and *Wheaties*. These are many of the foods I eat.

Bob Green's website states that he only gives his seal to companies that show a commitment to improving their nutritional profile. His website explains that a healthy lifestyle is within your reach and it's you that has to make the commitment to eat right and exercise. I really like that! Oprah wrote the Forward, which tells you something. If there's anyone who understands the challenges of weight loss, eating right and is a proponent of healthy living, it's Oprah. Bottom line, I eat most of the foods Bob Green endorses!

Examples of Products to Avoid

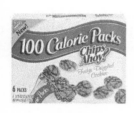

Kraft Foods, the parent company of *Nabisco*, states that *"Nabisco 100 Calorie Packs* are a great choice for those who want to snack and stay on track with their balanced eating routine." I know that many of you may be tempted to add these, or any of the other 19 available 100 calorie snacks into your diet, so let's examine exactly what you're getting for 100 calories.

You're getting exactly 0.81 ounces (23 grams) of product. That works out to a calorie density (CD) of 4.35. You'll recall from Chapter 19 that anything above a 3.1 CD is considered very high-calorie. The label tells me this is a "sensible solution" and is "low saturated fat" since it only contains three grams of total fat. While three grams of total fat might be acceptable in 16 ounces of soup (two servings), it sure is no bargain for less than an ounce of food product.

Okay, I've read what Madison Avenue wants me to know about the *Chips Ahoy 100 Calorie Pack*. Now let's see what its Nutrition Facts label and Ingredients List have to say. Besides the obvious 100 calories (25 from fat), I can see that I'm getting 0.5 grams of saturated fat and 2.5 of poly and monounsaturated fat. As you'll recall, these poly and monounsaturated fats are the omega-6 fats that are way out of balance in our diets due to the prevalence of processed foods like these 100 calorie packs.

Looking at the Ingredients List, the first ingredient is enriched flour, which is, of course, a refined grain that will temporarily spike our blood sugar causing us to be hungry before our next mealtime. The second ingredient is semisweet chocolate chips, which if you read the sub-ingredients in the parentheses, is really mostly sugar. The third ingredient is sugar again, followed by canola oil (omega-6), high fructose corn syrup (another added sugar), cornstarch, baking soda and salt.

The *Chips Ahoy 100 Calorie Pack* is a brilliant marketing idea and money-making product for *Nabisco*. It is not a brilliant food choice, nor part of either a healthy diet or something you even want to consider during a weight loss journey. In short, this is exactly the opposite of what you want to be eating since it has no real nutritional value. Save your 100 calories for something like a handful of grapes that will provide four-five times the weight (about four ounces), along with satiety and real nutrients. The grapes are not only better for you, but in my opinion they taste better and they will make you feel a whole lot better too.

Immunity Boosters

Although I've already discussed antioxidants in Chapter 22, I'd be remiss if I didn't warn you about all the "immunity boosting" claims that are advertised on food labels. Once again, as soon as food manufacturers figured out that you were interested in strengthening your immune system, they jumped right onto the band wagon. Every product from frozen vegetables to drinks now claims to "support," "enhance" or "boost" your immune system. These, as we now know, are structure and function claims that won't hold up when you compute the actual nutrition.

If there really were hard evidence to support these claims, the manufacturers would be petitioning the FDA and making much stronger health claims. To date, the only evidence that we can "enhance" the immune system with any form of supplement comes from studies with very old (my Mom says I should say elderly) and frail people. Researchers believe these supplements can be effective because elderly folks have immune systems that are starting to shut down.

Here's the real story. Study after study has proven that the only way to "boost" your immune system is to exercise. An interesting fact is that the effect of exercise on your immune system is very short-lived. Think hours, versus days or weeks. For those of us that take this health stuff seriously, we start to see an irrefutable pattern emerge. Eat right and exercise! There is no quick fix. You can't outsource your weight loss or buy good health for any amount of money.

Spending $30 - $50 for immunity enhancing supplements or drinks and powders may make you feel better about taking care of your health (think placebo effect). But while they probably won't hurt you, they won't really improve your health or help you lose weight. At best, these supplements are imitating vitamins at three to five times the cost (that's why they offer free shipping). At worst, these "immunity boosters" are just filling you with expensive, calorie-laden drinks. Bottom line, don't fall for any of these misleading and often, downright false, claims. Save your calories and dollars for real food.

Endorsements

Another thing you need to be aware of is the claim of "scientifically proven" or "doctor endorsed." Many products these days carry endorsements by so-called doctors, which may lead us to believe they are as good as prescriptions from our family physicians. Once again, most of these products have flimsy structure and function claims with outrageous price tags.

Many products claim that a certain doctor conducted 30 years of tests that prove the value of what are invariably very expensive products. Of course, they never say where these studies were published, who reviewed them and if acceptable review standards were used (and I can't find them). My first reaction is to wonder why every legitimate doctor in America isn't prescribing this stuff if it does the amazing things claimed on the websites. I guess that should tell us something.

My research into many of these products showed that some of the endorsers often have a financial interest or are in some way related to the companies that produce them. What they don't realize is that the person buying their product could be someone like my sister. She was like many people who tried to improve their health via these quick fixes but instead wasted valuable time. I believe that with correct, common sense information backed up with valid research studies, my sister could have lost weight and lived a longer, healthier life.

I've given you just a few examples so that you know what to

look for in food labels and the claims product manufacturers can make legally. We all need to look critically at food packaging and check both the nutrition label and the list of ingredients. Remember, many of the foods that claim "no trans fat" will list hydrogenated or partially hydrogenated oils in the list of ingredients, telling you that the product does, in fact, have trans fat. After what I've learned, I put those foods back on the shelf.

You also now know the three different claims the FDA will allow food manufacturers to make and that there are different ways to spot the foods that are better for you. The *Whole Grains Council* and *Bestlife* are just two examples.

It's vitally important that you develop the ability to know what you're getting when you purchase a food product. More and more these days, the packaged offerings in the super-market have been so highly and thoroughly processed that they no longer resemble food or contain the nutrients your body needs (think 100 calorie packs). You will find and eat the foods that are best for you only by systematically educating yourself and understanding the myriad ways you are being influenced. Of course as you get more serious about your health (after you've lost all that weight), you'll find that you're eating less food that comes out of a box, can or other type of package.

Years ago, due to successful lobbying efforts in Washington, D.C., we Americans deconstructed whole foods into their basic good and bad nutrients. It's very hard for any official entity to come out and say, "eat less refined sugar / avoid high fructose corn syrup," because the extremely well-funded sugar and corn lobbying groups would never permit it. These days we are told to consume less sodium, eat more omega-3s and less saturated fat. Instead we should be told (but aren't) to eat less processed food (that contains high sodium), more fish (omega-3) and less meat (saturated fat). Yep, this is the world you live in.

Start thinking about how you define food and you might find that you don't need to use your new label reading skills as often. Yes, I've become an expert in label reading, but truth be told, most of my food doesn't have a label (think Green Light foods). If you want to maintain the weight you lose, you'll need to start thinking about food in a whole different light.

24

It Costs $$ to Eat Well

Sometime ago my wife told me, "You have no idea how expensive it is to eat the way you do." As she does nearly all of the food shopping, I assumed that she was probably right and decided that it would be important to find out why. What I learned was amazing.

> Early humans had no such dilemma. The only foods they could eat were natural, organic and nutrient rich.

I discovered that we are biologically no different from our early ancestors who were continually on a quest for life-sustaining calories. The difference is that today we can get calories from a wide variety of foods, some that are good for us and some not so good. Early humans had no such dilemma. The only foods they could eat were natural, organic and nutrient rich. The game they hunted produced life-sustaining, calorie-dense meat along with the associated saturated fat.

Fortunately for them, it came in small enough doses that it was more beneficial than harmful. Can you imagine if the only way you could eat meat is if you felled an antelope with a sharp rock on the end of a stick? Puts it into perspective, doesn't it? And remember, our ancestors had only water to drink.

Fast-forward to today and we can very easily satisfy our daily quest for calories with a stop at a fast food restaurant or convenience store on our way to work. Early man had no such luxury. I believe the main reasons that two-thirds of us are overweight are that high calorie-dense and generally unhealthful food is cheap and has a long shelf life. Additionally, in our 21st century environment, there is a huge disparity in cost between "calorie-dense" and "nutrient-dense" foods that significantly contributes to our obesity epidemic. Let me explain.

In today's world, economic realities have driven us to a food supply that is easily prepared in large quantities, contains inexpensive ingredients, doesn't spoil easily and is readily transportable. Unfortunately, that means our food tends to contain refined grains, high levels of fat, sugar (e.g., high fructose corn syrup) and sodium, which are the exact opposite of what we should be eating. These foods are also generally high in calories (calorie-dense).

Remember, your body is really not very different from that of early humans, so it thrives best on nutrient-dense foods such as fruits, vegetables and whole grains. However, you're hard-wired to want the most calorie-dense foods like the aforementioned antelope so you can store fat for the times when food becomes scarce (which doesn't happen for most of us). The problem with most nutrient-dense foods is that they usually have a short shelf life, spoil easily, require more care in transportation, generally require you to prepare them at home, and often require refrigeration. These all add tremendously to the cost.

Adam Drewnowski, PhD, Director of the Center for Public Health Nutrition at the University of Washington, conducted research to determine the cost of a 2,000 calorie daily diet. He found that a calorie-dense diet (macaroni and cheese, *Twinkies*, etc.) could cost as little as $3.52, while the same 2,000 calories of nutrient-dense food (fresh vegetables, fish, fruits, whole grains, etc.) would cost an astronomical $36.32. This is per person, per day! So, my wife is right....it really does cost more to eat a healthy diet!

> A calorie-dense diet (macaroni and cheese, etc.) could cost as little as $3.52, while the same 2,000 calories of nutrient-dense food (fresh vegetables, etc.) would cost an astronomical $36.32 per day.

The problem these days is threefold. One, we still have that deep-rooted quest for calories, so when we have a choice, we tend to go for the calorie-dense foods that are not good for us. Second, our cash-strapped wallets are helping us make these same bad choices. The $3.52 daily meal plan may be the only realistic choice for some people. Finally, our sedentary lifestyle is the third leg in the triad of elusive modern-day wellness.

> Food advertising is designed to stimulate our age-old desire for the most calorie-dense foods.

We also can't expect much help from the world around us. Food advertising is designed to stimulate our age-old desire for the most calorie-dense foods. Closely watch the ads on TV and in print and you see how they appeal to our most basic quest for calories. The advertising uses terms like "filling" and "satisfy." It has even gone as far as using tag lines like "Obey your thirst" (*Sprite*), and "Do what feels right" (*Wendy's*). The feel good comfort food they are selling is scratching that million-year old itch of ours.

Finally, our food manufacturers, fast food establishments and restaurants have learned how to combine salt, sugar and fat along with changes in temperature, taste and texture to make food nearly impossible to resist. Let's face it; it's hard to get as excited about green beans as it is about a hot fudge sundae. Look at the ingredients in a hot fudge sundae and you'll see how this works: ice cream (fat / sugar / cold), fudge (sugar / hot), whipped cream (sugar / fat) and nuts (crunchy / salty). Amazingly delicious, but it's not something early humans had access to and therefore (unfortunately), isn't what we should be eating. This is what you're up against in modern day America!

So what can we do? First, we need to acknowledge that we must develop the skills to buy healthy fare with available food dollars. *McDonald's* has made it incredibly fast, convenient and inexpensive to feed our kids a *Happy Meal*. But if we want to be good parents and prepare our offspring for a lifetime of good health and wellness, we need to find a way to feed our family as much healthy food as our budget allows. This can be a challenge for some of us.

The good news is that the very act of trying to lose weight should have most of us eating less, especially if the self-assessment process has identified us as a "How Much" eater. This could free up extra dollars for more nutritious, albeit more expensive food choices. If you burn 2,000 calories a day, you only need 1,500 nutrient-dense calories a day during a weight-loss journey. Nutrient-dense foods are generally very filling, contain fewer calories and are excellent choices when trying to lose weight.

> If you burn 2,000 calories a day, you only need 1,500 nutrient-dense calories a day during a weight-loss journey.

Getting smart on the best foods for your body should help you focus your supermarket buying and further stretch those scarce food dollars. We can buy seasonal fruits and vegetables, buy in bulk, frequent farmers' markets and other local food producers (the ones that are truly cheaper than the grocery store) or start a "Victory Garden" like our parents did to grow our own produce in the backyard. Although we only have a wooden deck at our backyard in Virginia, my wife still grows all her herbs and even tomatoes in pots.

Additionally, we need to acknowledge that we just can't eat like everyone else around us, eat whatever we want, or make food choices based solely on what we see advertised. We also can't make our food choices based on easy availability and low cost, as these foods tend to be calorie-dense and nutritionally poor choices. In many other developed counties, families spend a much greater proportion of their discretionary income on high quality, fresh food.

Here in America we need to evaluate whether we're doing a better job of supplying our children with electronic gadgets than with nutritious food. This isn't easy since you and your kids are bombarded relentlessly with advertisements for both unhealthy, cheap food and electronic gadgets. Both can diminish your budget for healthy food. You need to be on guard and choose healthier foods, regardless of the pleas of your easily influenced children. But you already know, you're going to get very little help in making the best choices for your family from the world around you. It's truly "you against the world."

> You're going to get very little help in making the best choices for your family from the world around you. It's truly "you against the world."

It was only after I realized that I was on my own that I took active steps to educate myself. Every day I see people really trying to improve their health and lose weight, but they're stymied by the misinformation on food labels, relentless marketing and the cost of a truly healthy diet. While we're all not born to be activists, we all need to demand a healthier food supply and better labeling laws.

As I write and research information for this book, the debate rages on about "sin taxes" on certain foods, especially sugared soft drinks. While a lot of ideas are being promoted, the best way to get unhealthy foods out of our food supply is to simply stop buying them. As consumers, we do have the power to refuse to buy unhealthy products. Economics drive everything in this country. I'm not keeping the fast food chains in business, nor do I support the manufacturers of high calorie, sugar-added soft drinks. Do you?

I urge you to subscribe to the *Nutrition Action Newsletter* published by the Center for Science in the Public Interest. Subscription info is in the Sources section of this book. Each month the newsletter provides the latest information on health, research studies and which foods available in your supermarket are the best for you. It has been an invaluable resource for me.

While the reality of this chapter may pose your biggest challenge, I'm convinced that a reasonably healthy diet and an appropriate weight for our height are within reach for all of us.

25

By the Numbers

In order to address the deteriorating physical condition of many Americans, the FDA has published and occasionally updates their recommendations for an average 2,000* calorie daily diet. The information below is their current advice for eating a healthy diet. It's important to note that the 2000 calorie diet was designed to maintain a healthy weight, but not necessarily to lose weight. Therefore on the chart below, the current advice from Uncle Sam is in bold and I've added my comments to help you lose weight.

> It's important to note that the 2000 calorie diet was designed to maintain a healthy weight, but not necessarily to lose weight.

FDA Recommendations for a Healthy Diet

Total Fat – 20-35 percent of calories. That's a maximum of 65 grams of fat per day (2,000 calorie daily diet*).

- I'd shoot for around 25-45 grams (approx. 20 percent) or fewer, especially if you have significant weight to lose. Cutting out fat can really help you achieve that 500 calorie difference between what you eat and what you burn.

---

* I refer often to a "2,000 calorie daily diet" since this number has become somewhat of a standard when talking about nutrition. You may or may not require this many calories per day. It's interesting to know that 50 years ago the average diet was closer to 3,000 calories owing to our more active lifestyle (mostly at work). Our current lifestyle simply does not require as many calories as it once did. Unfortunately, this comes at a time when the amount and variety of foods (and the calorie count) are the most abundant ever recorded in the USA. If you want to participate in some of those "fun" calories, you have to add a fair amount of movement to your daily routine. These days that means looking for opportunities to get exercise, whether it is in the gym or elsewhere.

<u>Saturated Fat</u> – **Less than 10 percent of calories, or 20 grams a day.**

- Shoot for 10 grams or fewer while you're actively losing weight. Remember, most of your fats should be monounsaturated (olive oil, nuts, etc.), polyunsaturated (omega-6) and omega-3 (fish, etc). Ratio should be 3:1 or three of omega-6 to one of omega-3. Your omega-6 fats are the oils in processed foods, so to get the correct ratio, eat less processed food and **more** omega-3 food. Note that meat is very high in **omega-6** and saturated fat.

<u>Trans Fat</u> – **As little as possible (defined as less than two grams per day).**

- Aim for zero! If you're really adept at spotting hydrogenated oils you could avoid all trans fat. Look for the words "hydrogenated" or "partially-hydrogenated" on any packaged food ingredients list. Do not depend on product labeling that says "Zero Trans Fat per Serving" as that food probably has trans fat.

<u>Fruits and Vegetables</u> – **Nine servings or more per day. That equals two (2) cups of fruit and two and a half (2.5) cups of vegetables each day.**

- These are the plant-based foods that you must eat to be healthy. Mom was right!

<u>Grains</u> – **Six or more servings a day; at least 25 grams. Half should be whole grains.**

- I'd try for 25-50 grams per day and aim for whole grains all the time, especially when eating bread. You'll get the less desirable refined grain in many cereals, pastas, crackers, etc. Look for "100% whole wheat" on the label to ensure you are eating whole grains. Caution: there're plenty of calories and sodium in bread, so go easy.

Sodium – Less than 2,400 milligrams (mgs) a day, 1,600 if you're middle-aged or older, have high blood pressure or are African American.

- You can slash your sodium intake markedly by choosing natural plant based (Green Light) foods instead of pre-packaged and processed foods. Unless you want to start using blood pressure medication in your early 40s, I'd aim for around 1,500 mg per day (American Heart Association recommendation).

Weight – Appropriate to your height with a Body Mass Index (BMI) below 25.

- See the BMI chart and my recommendations for a target weight for both men and women.

Physical Activity – 150 minutes (2.5 hours) per week of moderate intensity aerobic exercise and muscle-strengthening exercise two days per week.

- Many <u>healthy</u> people with a BMI under 25 get 60 minutes worth of physical activity three-four times a week. If you're trying to lose weight, you should exercise four-five times a week, even if like me, your self-assessment doesn't indicate that lack of exercise is a key contributor to your overweight condition.

I was already very active and still gaining weight, so while I didn't identify exercise as an important practice in my Guiding Star (see Chapter 27); I still made sure that I stayed active. Conversely, if you are not currently exercising and you want to achieve and maintain an appropriate weight for your height, you'll probably need to develop an exercise regimen.

It's not that hard to track the recommendations from the FDA for fats, sodium, grains, etc since they are printed on the label of any prepared food (now that you're a graduate of Label Reading 101). In time, you'll find that you use less food that comes out of a can or a box. When you eat fresh fruits and vegetables, you don't need to worry about sodium content or saturated fat (unless you add it).

For meat (saturated fat) that you prepare yourself, you can estimate once you know what a standard (generally four-ounce) serving looks like and contains. It's about the size of your fist. I still limit myself to 50-60 grams of fat per day, but here is the foot stomper: I get most of my fat grams from polyunsaturated and monounsaturated fats. They're the fats in non-stick margarine, vegetable oil, nuts, fish, olive oil, etc. You should have very little fat from saturated and trans fats in a healthy diet! We need fat in our diet, but not the saturated and trans fat that are in so many of our (Red Light) foods.

A lower sodium number will be the hardest to achieve. Check out the sodium content in any prepared food item (anything that comes out of a box, bag or can). Check even if you add fresh ingredients like meat and veggies. Look especially at soups and prepared pasta dishes. Multiply the per-serving sodium number times the total servings and then divide by the real number of servings for you and your family.

> Reducing the sodium in your diet will be the hardest to achieve.

Many products indicate they have 600 milligrams of sodium per serving and contain five small servings. Realistically assuming that there are four adequate servings would mean 3,000 mgs of sodium total divided by four, or 750 grams for each person for just that item. Often, you'll go right past 1,500 mgs in a single meal—the number many of us should limit ourselves to for an entire day. Americans consume way too much salt! If you have high blood pressure, limiting your sodium is just as important as losing weight.

Don't be discouraged if you are not a numbers person and don't like to keep track of calories or milligrams of sodium. I never did. It is important however, to understand how the nutrition makeup of any given food choice will affect your progress on a weight-loss journey. Just realizing how much sodium was in prepared foods steered me toward foods that not only had less sodium, but also were lower in calories.

> Americans consume way too much salt! If you have high blood pressure, limiting your sodium is just as important as losing weight.

As I educated myself on the FDA standards for healthy eating, I was able to use that information for both weight loss and an improved diet. It wasn't always necessary to determine how much of a food I'd consume, but to know if I'd be better off choosing something else. In many cases, that's precisely what I did. For example, when invited to a backyard BBQ (where there were no Nutrition Facts Labels), I chose a barbecued chicken breast instead of bratwurst.

Bottom Line: I never counted calories, sodium, or anything during my weight loss journey. But the understanding of how much, or in the case of fat, how little I should consume steered me towards the Green Light foods I enjoy today.

26

Lose 30 Pounds in 30 Weeks

> By recording your weight each Friday, you'll know when you're getting it right. The scale doesn't lie!

Once you've worked your way through the Self-Assessment and assimilated the Five Basic Truths, you can start the trial-and-error process of getting your body back into balance. By recording your weight each Friday, you'll know when you're getting it right. The scale doesn't lie! While you can fluctuate as much as five pounds either way due to hydration, if you're watching your sodium (salt) intake, you'll see less fluctuation in your weekly weight.

Many people ask me how often they should weigh themselves. I suggest once a week (every Friday morning) as I explained above if you're on a weight loss journey. You'll drive yourself crazy if you weigh yourself more often. Once you've achieved an appropriate weight for your height, you should weigh yourself every day. That way you'll know immediately when you've put on a pound or two and can take action to get back to your target weight.

My personal "Rubicon" is 173 pounds, and unlike Caesar, when I cross it, I come right back. I do this by switching gears between eating the same number of calories that I burn each day to that all important 500 calorie deficit. It's a skill I mastered long ago (you will too), and in less than a couple week's time (generally) I'm back at my target weight!

A simple way to record your weight each week during your journey is illustrated in the following chart. Remember, the only way you'll know that your efforts are paying off is when you see progress week after week. It took a long time to put on that weight, and in spite of what the commercial weight-loss world promises, it's going to take some time to take it off.

If you lose about one pound a week (average) you will be doing very well! You'll be losing it in a healthy way that won't make your body rebel or sick. And most importantly, you'll be able to sustain the weight loss when you reach your ideal BMI and weight.

To remind you, keep a chart like the one on the following page where you keep the scale. Or, use a calendar to record your weight.

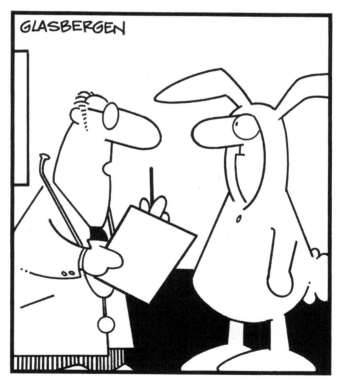

**"If hopping burns more calories than walking,
and it helps you eat more salad, then OK,
I approve of the Bunny Suit Diet."**

Lose 30 Pounds in 30 Weeks

Date _____ Weight _____   Date _____ Weight _____

Date _____ Weight _____   Date _____ Weight _____

Date _____ Weight _____   Date _____ Weight _____

Date _____ Weight _____   Date _____ Weight _____

Date _____ Weight _____   Date _____ Weight _____

Date _____ Weight _____   Date _____ Weight _____

Date _____ Weight _____   Date _____ Weight _____

Date _____ Weight _____   Date _____ Weight _____

Date _____ Weight _____   Date _____ Weight _____

Date _____ Weight _____   Date _____ Weight _____

Date _____ Weight _____   Date _____ Weight _____

Date _____ Weight _____   Date _____ Weight _____

Date _____ Weight _____   Date _____ Weight _____

Date _____ Weight _____   Date _____ Weight _____

Date _____ Weight _____   Date _____ Weight _____

27

Tying It All Together

Even though this is a fairly straightforward book, it has a lot of information for you to absorb. I'd suggest that you keep this book handy for reference during your weight-loss journey. You'll need to continually refer to this information to help train yourself in the basic concepts of weight loss and discover what works for you. But what should you do first? How do you get started?

> The most important advice, however, is that you must take ownership of your own weight loss journey.

A wise man once said that a journey of 10,000 miles begins with a single step. That is a good mind-set to have, especially if you have significant weight to lose. The most important advice, however, is that you must take ownership of your own weight loss journey. As the title of this book states, "You Can't Outsource Weight Loss..." or throw any amount of money at your weight problem. Only by identifying how you gained the excess weight and then addressing those specific areas will you be able to permanently lose weight.

The young woman mentioned earlier in the book who identified herself as a "Why" eater wouldn't have lost weight if she used the same practices that I, as a "What" eater, did. In fact, I don't think she would've been successful at all if she hadn't started with the self-assessment process. I mention it only because I want to reinforce the overall concept of this book. **Only you can determine which practices explained in this book will work for you.**

> Only by identifying how you gained the excess weight and then addressing those specific areas will you be able to permanently lose weight.

> You must be willing to engage your thought process to be successful in a weight loss journey.

I know that you want me to tell you exactly what you must do to succeed at losing weight. That is, in fact, the formula for writing many of the thousands of other weight loss books. But this book is different; it's about you taking control to learn how to successfully lose weight and keep it off. Many of my friends who know how knowledgeable I am on the subject ask me to give them the CliffsNotes on weight loss. While CliffsNotes work great for *The Catcher in the Rye*, the same approach simply won't work for weight loss!

The key to successful permanent weight loss is taking the time, whether days or weeks, for your self-assessment, learning the Five Basic Truths and then testing the practices through trial and error. You must be willing to engage your thought process to be successful in a weight loss journey. Just as exercising wasn't the key for me to lose weight, some of the information and practices in this book (although legitimate and valuable) may not be the key for you.

Many people look at me quizzically when I say that there'll be a period of trial and error. However, every single person I've ever spoken to who's succeeded in permanent weight loss has described a similar journey of self-discovery and personal involvement. So simply stated, don't assume everything you try will work, that you'll get it right the first time, or what worked for a friend or spouse will be right for you.

I ran into the young lady I have mentioned throughout the book more than two years after she told me that my seminar "changed her life." She confidently said that she lost an additional 20 pounds and was now a very svelte 5'6", approximately 120-pound young woman. She clearly has implemented many, if not most, of the skills outlined in this book. While she didn't mention it specifically, I'd bet that after she learned to eat for the right reasons, she also learned to eat the right foods. Many people "stair-step" their way through a weight loss journey, first addressing the root cause of their overweight condition, then use their new-found knowledge of calorie density, drink choices, sleep, etc. to eat more nutritiously, live a healthier life and achieve an optimum weight.

> You must make lifestyle changes to achieve permanent weight loss!

Don't underestimate the power of learned behavior. Although you shouldn't make changes that you can't do forever, you'll see how easy it is to fall back into eating and living as you previously did. You'll remember that I shared that I'd pop food in my mouth unconsciously and then have to spit it out when I realized I was eating the wrong kind of foods. You must make lifestyle changes to achieve permanent weight loss!

Like exercise, a go-slow process is necessary when you begin a weight-loss journey. If at first you try too hard and fail, it'll be far too easy to just give up. I started with very small changes to my diet, at first just with my drink choices. When I realized sleep was a key factor, I successfully added an extra half hour to each night's sleep. I was encouraged when I started to make progress and eagerly attempted other changes. Experimentation, or trial and error, are critical steps in a weight loss journey.

Your biggest challenge will be to find and sustain that delicate balance of eating well, enjoying your food and still achieving a 500-calorie a day deficit. Remember, once you achieve permanent weight loss, you can add back those 500 calories each day. I hope you discover, as I did, that eating the same amount of calories that you burn each day is something you can do forever.

> Experimentation, or trial and error, are critical steps in a weight loss journey.

Not everything worked for me or was even doable. I thought about giving up pizza and wine, but quickly realized that wouldn't work

> I thought about giving up pizza and wine, but quickly realized that wouldn't work for me.

for me. Again, this will be a trial-and-error period and if you're listening to your body, you'll know when you're getting it right. If listening to your body seems like too much of a touchy-feely concept, remember, I'm a *Myers Briggs Type Indicator* ESTJ who flew Navy jets for the past 28 years. If I could learn to listen to my body, trust me, you can too!

To help you get started, I've created a diagram called "Your Guiding Star" to help you focus your efforts. This is a way for you to identify and record the top five practices that work for you. As you complete the Self-Assessment process, start to populate the five points of the star. Yes, you always can change the points as you get smarter and discover practices that are more suited to your situation.

My points started simply with just drink choices, followed by sleep. When I discovered I was a "What" eater, I learned that choosing low calorie-dense foods really helped me lose weight. I've included many different concepts in this book because I know what worked for me won't necessarily work for everyone.

To complete your personal Guiding Star, you'll need to address such varied factors as sleep, calorie density, drink choices, stress, sodium, exercise, fats, the glycemic index and the ability to accurately read food labels (so you'll know what you're eating). You'll have a holistic approach of returning your body back into balance by combining your top five points. My five points worked for me, but you can include anything helpful, even a practice not listed above if it helps you achieve permanent weight loss.

Ed's Guiding Star

1. Make better **Drink Choices**. More water or drink lower calorie beverages.

2. Get **More Sleep**.

3. Make better **Food Choices**.
   • Stoplight Chart
   • Calorie Density
   • Glycemic Index

4. **Reduce my Stress** with exercise, goal setting and quiet time.

5. **Reward myself**. Pizza and wine on Friday night.

Write your personal Guiding Star practices clockwise, from "1" to "5," with "1" being the easiest to implement, and then add on the others as you discover what works best. This, I believe, is the most successful approach. Don't forget "Reward" as a possibility for your fifth and final practice. Relaxing with a couple of slices of pepperoni pizza and a glass of wine on Friday night was my way of rewarding myself for the results I saw on the scale that morning.

Your Guiding Star

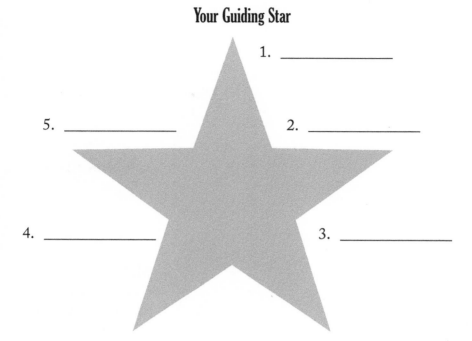

1. _____

2. _____

3. _____

4. _____

5. _____

Finally, as adults trying to learn a foreign language realize, it's only after you start dreaming in the new language that you know you're starting to get it. This may occur for you when you put together all the pieces of weight loss. You'll catch yourself unconsciously making the right choices and wake up one morning realizing that you're on the road to permanent weight loss. For some people, the effect is even more powerful. I met several people, mostly "Why" eaters, who succeeded to the point that they realized they were finally free from a life enslaved to food. Can you imagine that for yourself?

Losing weight was one of the most liberating and exciting evolutions in my entire life. I've flown in combat, commanded a squadron and landed on an aircraft carrier at night, but nothing compares to the satisfaction of having achieved something that eludes so many Americans: Permanent weight loss! Yes, it'll take some, perhaps a lot of effort, but you can do it and you'll be amazed when the "new you" (no matter your age) emerges.

I know you can do it! Please tell me about your successful weight loss journey via email at my website, www.YouCant OutsourceWeightLoss.com.

The Body Mass Index (BMI) Chart

Weight / Height	100	105	110	115	120	125	130	135	140	145	150	155	160	165	170	175	180	185	190	195	200	205	210	215	220	225	230	235	240	245	250
5'0"	20	21	21	22	23	24	25	26	27	28	29	30	31	32	33	34	35	36	37	38	39	40	41	42	43	44	45	46	47	48	49
5'1"	19	20	21	22	23	24	25	26	26	27	28	29	30	31	32	33	34	35	36	37	38	39	40	41	42	43	43	44	45	46	47
5'2"	18	19	20	21	22	23	24	25	26	27	27	28	29	30	31	32	33	34	35	36	37	37	38	39	40	41	42	43	44	45	46
5'3"	18	19	19	20	21	22	23	24	25	26	27	27	28	29	30	31	32	33	34	35	35	36	37	38	39	40	41	42	43	43	44
5'4"	17	18	19	20	21	21	22	23	24	25	26	27	27	28	29	30	31	32	33	33	34	35	36	37	38	39	39	40	41	42	43
5'5"	17	17	18	19	20	21	22	22	23	24	25	26	27	27	28	29	30	31	32	32	33	34	35	36	37	37	38	39	40	41	42
5'6"	16	17	18	19	19	20	21	22	23	23	24	25	26	27	27	28	29	30	31	31	32	33	34	35	36	36	37	38	39	40	40
5'7"	16	16	17	18	19	20	20	21	22	23	23	24	25	26	27	27	28	29	30	31	31	32	33	34	34	35	36	37	38	38	39
5'8"	15	16	17	17	18	19	20	21	21	22	23	24	24	25	26	27	27	28	29	30	30	31	32	33	33	34	35	36	36	37	38
5'9"	15	16	16	17	18	18	19	20	21	21	22	23	24	24	25	26	27	27	28	29	30	30	31	32	32	33	34	35	35	36	37
5'10"	14	15	16	16	17	18	19	19	20	21	22	22	23	24	24	25	26	27	27	28	29	29	30	31	32	32	33	34	34	35	36
5'11"	14	15	15	16	17	17	18	19	20	20	21	22	22	23	24	24	25	26	27	27	28	29	29	30	31	31	32	33	33	34	35
6'0"	14	14	15	16	16	17	18	18	19	20	20	21	22	22	23	24	24	25	26	26	27	28	28	29	30	31	31	32	33	33	34
6'1"	13	14	15	15	16	16	17	18	18	19	20	20	21	22	22	23	24	24	25	26	26	27	28	28	29	30	30	31	32	32	33
6'2"	13	13	14	15	15	16	17	17	18	19	19	20	21	21	22	22	23	24	24	25	26	26	27	28	28	29	30	30	31	31	32
6'3"	12	13	14	14	15	16	16	17	17	18	19	19	20	21	21	22	22	23	24	24	25	26	26	27	27	28	29	29	30	31	31
6'4"	12	13	13	14	15	15	16	16	17	18	18	19	19	20	21	21	22	23	23	24	24	25	26	26	27	27	28	29	29	30	30

The BMI Chart is very simple to use, plus there are many online versions that are very useful. Start on the left had vertical column and find your height. This chart is for both men and women, and while not perfect, it's universally accepted as a gauge for how appropriate your height and weight are for good health.

Once you have your height, move right through the body of the chart to the box that falls under your weight (at top). At 5'11" and 170 pounds, I'm at a BMI of 24 (in the lightly shaded (healthy) section of the BMI chart). Any BMI that is under 25 and above 18 is fantastic.

You Can't Outsource Weight Loss… But You Can Lose Weight and Be Thin Forever!

Exercise Startup Checklist and Log

✓ Checklist

- ❑ Clearance from Doctor to begin an exercise program
- ❑ Comfortable and safe footwear and season appropriate / loose fitting clothing
- ❑ Warm-up (moving all limbs to get the blood flowing) Use elliptical on low setting
- ❑ Cardio (brisk walking, treadmill, exercise bike, elliptical or stair-stepper
- ❑ Resistance work / light weight lifting
- ❑ Stretching / cool down

Sample Log

Date	Warm-up	Cardio	Weight/Resistence		Stretch/ Cool Down
	Exercise: Time:	Exercise: Time:	Exercise: Reps: Exercise: Reps:	Exercise: Reps: Exercise: Reps:	❑
	Exercise: Time:	Exercise: Time:	Exercise: Reps: Exercise: Reps:	Exercise: Reps: Exercise: Reps:	❑
	Exercise: Time:	Exercise: Time:	Exercise: Reps: Exercise: Reps:	Exercise: Reps: Exercise: Reps:	❑

Daily Meal Log

	What + how much food I ate	Why I ate these	How I felt	How much I moved
Date				
Breakfast				
Lunch				
Dinner				
Snack				
Date				
Breakfast				
Lunch				
Dinner				
Snack				
Date				
Breakfast				
Lunch				
Dinner				
Snack				

You Can't Outsource Weight Loss… But You Can Lose Weight and Be Thin Forever!

Daily Meal Log

	What + how much food I ate	Why I ate these	How I felt	How much I moved
Date				
Breakfast				
Lunch				
Dinner				
Snack				
Date				
Breakfast				
Lunch				
Dinner				
Snack				
Date				
Breakfast				
Lunch				
Dinner				
Snack				

Daily Meal Log

	What + how much food I ate	Why I ate these	How I felt	How much I moved

Date_____

Breakfast				
Lunch				
Dinner				
Snack				

Date_____

Breakfast				
Lunch				
Dinner				
Snack				

Date_____

Breakfast				
Lunch				
Dinner				
Snack				

You Can't Outsource Weight Loss... But You Can Lose Weight and Be Thin Forever!

Acknowledgments

Any project of this magnitude requires many dedicated and talented people behind the scenes to support the efforts of the guy whose name appears on the front cover. I would like to thank RADM Tony Cothron, USN (Ret), for not only taking the time to attend my very first Wellness Seminar, but for critiquing my performance afterwards. A career Navy Intelligence Officer, he taught me that to be effective, the delivery is as important as the message. My seminars to this day incorporate his sage advice.

Thanks to Randy Glasbergen, one of the country's most talented and beloved cartoonists for his funny and oftentimes deadly serious cartoons. See all of Randy's cartoons at www. glasbergen.com. Thanks also to Ken Kropkowski, of the "ken" Group, LLC for teaching me the value of "vibrating your network."

To the talented women that helped with this book project: I can't say enough for how much you improved my original vision for the book, but also the final manuscript and packaging. Donna Giannola did a great job on the Bluewater Health Concepts Logo, one that I am proud to represent my company and the concept of living well in modern day America. I thank Janet Ratzlaff for her superb job of proofreading the manuscript, expertly providing proper English and grammar while preserving what I hope is an easily read and understood message. Any errors in the final product are due to me making additions subsequent to her fine work.

The cover and book design were masterfully created by Karla Hills of KKCreativeSolutions.com Art Direction & Graphic Design, after she received no more input than the title of the book. Those who know me can see how this cover is a perfect match for my personality and presentation style. Special thanks to my dear friend and mentor, Deedee Collins who not only read the manuscript and offered many ideas for improvement, but also provided superb career advice that has served me well since retiring from the Navy.

To Ida Halasz, whom I can't thank enough and who ultimately coordinated this entire book project. I met Ida while still on active duty and she agreed to sign on to this project from the very beginning. Ida is what every first-time author needs—someone to guide them through the whole process from start to finish. Ida has been a superb coach, mentor, editor, advisor, coordinator, savvy business partner, career coach and ultimately a friend. Ida, you know I could not have done this without you and I appreciate not only the many hours you spent on this project, but also for your passion and commitment for healthy living.

To my wife Debra, and sons Ed and Jean-Marc, I can't thank you enough for the support you have given me during this entire project. You all gave up a great deal of time with me so that I could dedicate my energies towards writing this book. Without your love and encouragement, this book would never have been completed.

And finally, to my sister Michelle. Your death was the catalyst to write this book and hopefully help others to achieve a life of true wellness and happiness. Rest in peace.

Sources

Much of the information in this book can be found in numerous sources and multiple places on the Internet. If the information is widely accepted as true (like exercise is good for the human body), then no source is noted. The genesis of this book was clearly my sister's death, but the motivation to write it came after I realized how hard it was for the average person to find accurate information on permanent weight loss. The key for this book was for me to wade through all the incorrect and misleading information that is touted in the weight loss world and only include the information that really helps to lose weight.

The studies I reference throughout the text and list in this section are all from respected sources and have been subject to peer review. Either the specific information is presented or the web link is provided. While you can't outsource weight loss, you can be subjected to some fairly flimsy claims in many weight loss books. I have worked hard to just present you the facts in order to achieve permanent weight loss. I've stressed throughout the book that your engagement in the process is vital for success. Information that is my own opinion, or based on observation / discussion at Wellness Seminars is either mentioned in the text or annotated in this section as such.

Chapter 1 – "The Facts" is a compilation of many different sources. The actual annual cost of health care and the sub-set of obesity related health care costs are widely disputed, probably because the number is so astronomical. Additionally, any discussion of obesity related costs (both medical and absenteeism related) can be viewed by some as participating in discriminatory behavior. My best source came from Leade Health Inc. and a white paper titled, "The Business Case for Weight/Obesity Management Using Health Coaching Interventions."

Most of the figures I use were derived from this paper which addresses the impact of obesity on workplace productivity and medical costs. This paper must be purchased, but is available online at www.leadehealth.com. Another valuable resource, although their numbers differ, is "The Relationship of Body Mass Index, Medical Costs, and Job Absenteeism by Timothy Bungum, DrPH; Monica Satterwhite, MS; Allen W. Jackson, EdD, James R. Morrow Jr, PhD available online at: http://www.atypon-link.com/PNG/doi/pdf/10.5555/ajhb.2003.27.4.456?cookieSet=1.

Thanks to David Rebich at the US Department of the Treasury for providing the information on Medicare costs and to Wikipedia for providing the explanation of the Present Value of the 75-year Actuarial Projections for Medicare costs.

Chapter 2 – "Five Basic Truths" are what I discovered during my own personal weight loss journey. While I have seen some of the individual truths in whole, or in part, in my research, the concept that you must understand all Five Basic Truths and assimilate them prior to starting your weight loss journey, is my own.

Chapters 3, 4, 5, 7, 8 – "Self-Assessment" is an important skill for many aspects of an individual's life, but it is a critical second step in the weight loss process (after you assimilate the Five Basic Truths). Many so called "Diets" recommend the keeping of a log or journal and I found this exercise a very valuable part of my self-assessment process. The idea for the "What, Why & How Times 2" came from my wife's January 2008 issue of Good Housekeeping magazine. While I had long ago discovered that I was a "What" eater, I intuitively knew that it couldn't be the same for everyone.

The sub-title of the Good Housekeeping article, written by Kate Torgovink states "It's not <u>what</u> you eat," and her excellent article, aimed at "Why" eaters, explains the value of keeping a food journal. With two known types, I was determined to discover if there were others. Through observation, interviews, and the feedback from seminar participants, I became convinced that we all fall predominantly, into at least one of the 4 categories described.

Chapter 6 – I'm a "Why" or Emotional Eater, so What can I do about it? The internet is full of explanations for emotional eating and the "triggers" that cause it. Some are better than others. I have included what I have <u>seen</u> as the top 10 triggers of emotional eating. Additionally, the "Mommy Syndrome" as well as "The Relationship from Hell' and "The Addict" are also based on my personal observations.

There is a lot of common sense information out there concerning emotional eating and what to do about it, the key is to determine if you are a garden variety emotional eater or if you actually have an eating disorder. As I mention in the text, this is the one area where you may need to engage professional counsel, and the EAT-26 and SCOFF Eating Disorder Quiz are good places to start. Also see the excellent discussion on eating disorders at About.com, <u>http://adam.about.com/reports/Eating-disorders.htm</u>.

Chapter 9 – "I'm Overweight, So What" was included because of the number of people that I have met that view being overweight as an undesirable, yet normal, human physical attribute. As we now know, it is not. The information concerning how many calories our Paleolithic ancestors burned while they hunted and gathered as compared to early farmers and those of us today, comes from the late anthropologist Marvin Harris of the University of Florida.

The information on cancer risk comes from the World Cancer Research Fund and was based on the analysis of more than 7,000 cancer studies. It's a behemoth 360 page report, but you can see their latest information at <u>www.dietandcancerreport.org</u>.

Chapter 10 – "Losing Weight - The Basics" is a conglomeration of many widely available mathematical formulas for losing weight. A very helpful resource was the original *Step-By-Step Diet Guide* that was previously a free download at www.BeachBody.com. Now you have to join to get access to it, but it is a good site to join if your assessment has identified you as someone who needs to exercise more or address food choices.

Also see Otto Kroger Associates at www.typetalk.com for information on how your personality type (MBTI) affects your ability to lose weight. Also look for the paper "Fat is a Typological Issue" by Janet Thuesen and Otto Kroeger.

Chapter 11 – "It's Five O'clock Somewhere," a song made famous (originally) by Jimmy Buffet, and more recently by Alan Jackson, was selected to remind us that we have to address today's drink choices, as well as food, if we are to achieve an appropriate weight for our height. There are literally thousands of sources out there but I thought Barry M. Popkin (and associates) and the Beverage Guidance Panel were the absolute best. Their paper "A New Proposed Guidance System for beverage Consumption in the United States" provided a great deal of the source material for this chapter and is available on line at http://www.ajcn.org/cgi/content/full/83/3/529?maxtoshow=&HITS=10&hits=10&RESULTFORMAT=1&andorexacttitle=and&titleabstract=A+New+Proposed+Guidance+System+for+Beverage+Consumption+in+the+United+States+&andorexacttitleabs=and&andorexactfulltext=and&searchid=1&FIRSTINDEX=0&sortspec=relevance&resourcetype=HWCIT. The June 2006 issue of *Nutrition Action Health Letter* does a great job of distilling what is a fairly technical paper and includes an interview with Dr. Popkin.

Another good resource was the survey published by the American Journal of Preventive Medicine in Oct 2004 titled "Changes in Beverage Intake Between 1977 and 2001" by

Samara Joy Nielsen, BS & Barry M. Popkin, PhD. You can buy the paper, as I did, or find it for free at: http://www.cpc.unc.edu/Plone/projects/nutrans/publications/Beverage%20trends-BP-Samara%202004.pdf.

The information on the different mechanisms for thirst and hunger comes from an article by Dr. Popkin titled "Global Dimensions of Sugary Beverages and Programmatic and Policy solutions" found in the CMR eJournal at: http://www.cardiometabolic-risk.org/cmrejournal/articles/vol2/v2i2a2.php.

Also see Barry M. Popkin's excellent book *"The World Is Fat — The Fads, Trends, Policies, and Products That Are Fattening The Human Race."* New York: Avery-Penguin Group, 2008.

The recommendation to drink only 10-15% of your calories each day can be found in numerous places on the Internet, including a September 2006 Indian Health Services publication titled the "Healthy Beverages Community Action Kit." This paper contains nearly identical recommendations for drink choices, but the best I can tell is that the 10-15% recommendation originated in the March 2006 edition of the American Journal of Clinical Nutrition.

The study referred to that reported a correlation between diet sodas and metabolic syndrome was titled "Dietary Intake and the Development of the Metabolic Syndrome. The Atherosclerosis Risk in Communities Study." This paper was published by the American Heart Association January 2008 by Pamela L. Lutsey, MPH, Lyn M. Steffen, PhD, MPH, RD, and June Stevens, PhD, MS, RD all from the Division of Epidemiology and Community Health, University of Minnesota, School of Public Health, Minneapolis, and the Department of Nutrition, University of North Carolina, Chapel Hill. Find it at: http://circ.ahajournals.org/cgi/content/abstract/CIRCULATIONAHA.107.716159v1.

The link between artificial sweeteners in diet drinks and hunger comes from eight years of data collected by Sharon P.

Fowler, MPH and her colleagues at the University of Texas Health Center, San Antonio. Find the information at: http://sci.tech-archive.net/Archive/sci.med.nutrition/2005-06/msg01172.html. My recommendation for daily drink choices are exactly what I have been drinking for six years now, and I suspect that of many healthy individuals. It is also pretty darn close to what Barry Popkin and his associates recommend in the papers referenced above.

Chapter 12 – "Alcohol" was included as I have seen how much the consumption of alcoholic beverages can affect both healthy living and the ability to achieve an appropriate weight for your height. Sources for this chapter include information from the Harvard School of Public Health (standard for daily alcohol consumption), The Women's Health Study and The Hutchison Study as quoted in the text. The 2010 conference in Barcelona, Spain info came from an Associated Press article as reported on Cleveland.com at http://www.cleveland.com/healthfit/index.ssf/2010/03/more_exercise_less_food_could.html.

Chapter 13 – "Exercise" was principally derived from my experiences and training during my 28 years in the US Navy. During my time in the service, we truly became a culture of fitness and the Navy provided many talented exercise instructors at our base gyms that taught me what I share with you in this chapter. The instructors are too many to name individually, but they are collectively responsible for the common-sense approach I take towards exercise to this day.

Chapter 14 – "Sodium" The 150,000 deaths per year figure was adapted from the National High Blood Pressure Education Program as reported in the Jan 2004 American Journal of Public Health. It stated that if we could reduce the sodium in our diets by 20 percent that it would result in 150,000 fewer American deaths. The recommendations for sodium intake can vary depending on who's giving you advice.

The absolute best, 2-page, easy to read discussion on sodium intake comes from a USDA Center for Nutrition Policy and Promotion paper co-authored by Doctors Etta Saltos and Shanthy Bowman in May 1997. The paper is titled "Dietary Guidance On Sodium: Should We Take It With A Grain Of Salt?" This was the USDAs response to a TV network report that criticized Federal Government recommendations to eat less salt. Not only does the paper address the poor methodology of a study (published by the Journal of the American Medical Association) that claimed "people with normal blood pressure" need not worry about reducing sodium, but it contains 3 very useful figures detailing sodium intake by sex and race, and food group contribution. This is also one of the sources where I found the figure that 75% of the sodium we consume is added during food processing. Download this very informative paper at: http://www.cnpp.usda.gov/publications/nutritioninsights/insight3.pdf.

Recommendations for daily sodium intake as stated in the text are fairly consistent between the medical establishment and US Government Agencies. Trying to nail down what our current national average for daily sodium intake was harder to accomplish. This is due to the variances in men (4,178mg) and women (2,933mg) and differences in age and ethnic groups. I simply used an average (3,500mg) which is still way too much daily sodium for any of us.

Chapter 15 – "Sleep: Get Your ZZZZZs." There is an amazing amount of information out there concerning how important it is that we get sufficient sleep during a weight loss journey. Some of it is all over the map, but the bottom line remains that the lack of sleep will impede your weight loss efforts. Background information for this chapter came from the Nurses' Health Study which followed 68,163 women for 16 years, a randomized crossover clinical sleep study of 12 men at the University of Chicago that demonstrated the elevation of ghrelin and reduction in leptin levels when sleep deprived, and an excellent study of 1,024 participants in the population-based Wisconsin Sleep Cohort Study that associated proportional increased Body Mass Index with less than 8 hours sleep as reported by Patricia Prinz in "Sleep, Appetite, and Obesity – What Is the Link?" All available online for free.

Chapter 16 – "Stress" - WebMD has an excellent and informative archive article titled "Can Stress Cause Weight Gain?" available at http://www.webmd.com/diet/features/can-stress-cause-weight-gain that was a useful source, as was the Mayo Clinic's Dr. Edward T. Creagan article "How do I control stress-induced weight gain?" The symptoms of stress came primarily from Stress.com at http://www.symptoms-of-stress.com/. Many of the recommendations came from my personal experiences in dealing with stress during my Navy career.

Chapter 17 – "What Should I Weigh" and the "Target Weight" chart were included because of all the misleading information out there on what healthy individuals should weigh. There have been several studies claiming overweight people live longer that have garnered overwheling press coverage, if for no other reason than they'll know they will have a receptive US audience. One of the most widely published was a Canadian study in 2005 that said overweight people were 17 percent less likely to die than those of normal weight.

Even more famous was the 2007 Center for Disease Control (CDC) study that indicated overweight people had a "Slightly lower risk" of death than people of normal weight (defined as a BMI of 18.5-24.9). Never mind that a third of us are obese and most of the reporting failed to indicate that this group doesn't see the benefit.

Now there is an Australian study that says it is okay to be overweight (not obese), if you have made it as far as your seventies. The study does caution that it isn't a good thing to be overweight after 70 if you have diabetes, osteoarthritis, and I would assume heart disease, high blood pressure, etc. How many elderly Americans fit into this group? There is some (common sense) evidence in this study that indicates once you get into your seventies, and get sick, having a little extra fat reserves might carry you through a serious illness compared to someone who is at a very low BMI. All the studies can be found online, but I assume that if you have read this book, you're really thinking it is a good idea to achieve an appropriate weight for your height. Bravo!

The Nutritionist Standard for a healthy weight is 100 pounds for individuals 5 feet tall and then an additional 5 pounds for women, and 6 pounds for men, for every inch over 5 feet. Example – a 5' 11" man would be 166 pounds, while a 5' 6" female would be 130 pounds.

The recommendation for maximum waistline measurements for both men and women came from my AARP magazine, but I have seen it repeated all over the Internet and in many other respected publications as well.

My Target Weight chart gets challenged more than anything else at my seminars, but I know I have it right because virtually every individual I speak to was at the target weight for their height at some point in their early life. Sources as stated in the text were combined in a very unscientific formula to come up with the weights listed.

While I could have designed a Target Weight chart that showed weights more in line with our much lighter ancestors, I felt it was unrealistic with today's plentiful food supply to shoot for anything much less. Understand though, that while the weights listed are really on the top (heavier) end of the scale (average BMI of 21-24), if we all could collectively reach these weights it would have a dramatic effect on our health and would drastically lower national medical expenses.

Chapter 18 – "All Fats Are Not Created Equal" was sourced from information on the internet and the US Government recommendations for a healthy diet. The characterization of worst to best fats is my own opinion. The benefits we may realize from omega-3 and 6 fatty acids are all over the place and I have consolidated what seems to be the general consensus. I attempted to dig into some of the studies but realized that there is incontrovertible evidence that we all should have much less trans and saturated fat in our diet, and the fat we do get should be omega-3s and 6s in the right ratios.

This also compliments the idea that the key is to eat more like people did 10,000 years ago. The Conscious Life is also a great resource with a wonderful article that I recommend. See Anti-Inflammatory Diet: How to Balance omega-3 and omega-6 Fatty Acids at: http://theconsciouslife.com/anti-inflammatory-diet-how-to-balance-omega-3-omega-6-fats.htm.

The information on the study of Japanese men was by Dr. Akira Sekikawa (and associates) who is the Assistant Professor of Epidemiology at the Graduate School of Public Health at the University of Pittsburg. Results of the study were published in the *American Journal of Epidemiology*, January 22nd, 2007, and referenced in 5 August 2008 *Journal of the American College of Cardiology*. Find the full online study results at: http://aje.oxfordjournals.org/cgi/content/full/165/6/617.

There appears to be wide-spread agreement about the effect of increased omega-3 on improved cognitive function including a 2005 study, as reported in the European Journal of Clinical Investigation that indicated omega-3 supplements were also effective. The paper, titled "Cognitive and physiological effect of omega-3 polyunsaturated fatty acid supplementation in healthy subject" was written at the University of Siena, Siena, Italy and published in the European Journal of Clinical Investigation. http://www3.interscience.wiley.com/journal/118685041/abstract?CRETRY=1&SRETRY=0.

Chapter 19 – "Calorie Density – Eat More, Weigh Less." The internet is full of excellent advice about the best low calorie density foods and how water content and whole grains affect satiety. A very short, but information packed resource was the article by Shereen Jegtvig, titled Nutrient Density – "What Makes Superfoods So Super," available at About.com. Also see http://www.nutritiondata.com/topics/fullness-factor that has a very interesting graph that shows the satiety index of common foods. The actual calorie density numbers for the foods listed can vary from one resource to another and the numbers listed are representative of foods from low to high calorie density.

Another good source included Barbara Rolls. Energy Density and Nutrition in Weight Control Management. In The Permanente Journal, Spring 2003, Volume 7 No.2.

Also see http://www.wisegeek.com/what-does-200-calories-look-like.htm for photos of 200 calories of many popular foods.

Chapter 20 – The **Food Stoplight Charts** were adapted from (believe it or not) the Navy's guide to sexual harassment. Back when women were joining the war fighting ranks in large numbers, the Navy published a very successful guide to help identify sexual harassment with Red Light, Yellow Light and Green Light behavior. It was very simple, and when adapted for foods that can help or hurt us in losing weight it tested amazingly well. BeachBody.com has a similar, but more complex 5-part chart called "Michi's Ladder" available on-line.

Chapter 21 – "The Glycemic Index." The most useful resource for this chapter came from Mendosa.com http://www.mendosa.com/gilists.htm and David Mendosa's excellent explanation of both the Glycemic Index and Glycemic Load. His paper, the "Revised International Table of Glycemic Index (GI) and Glycemic Load (GL) Values" – 2008, not only has a very clear explanation of what the commercial weight loss programs have been touting, but it also contains what he describes as "the definitive table for both the GI and GL" for nearly 2,500 popular foods. The table in his article was provided by Professor Jennie Brand-Miller of the University of Sydney. The comparison of the GI and GL of watermelon comes from this paper.

The Glycemic Index figure (roller coaster) is my own based on both my understanding of the effects of high GI / GL foods and my observations of numerous individuals in an office environment. The benefits of a Low GI diet and How to Switch to a Low GI Diet come from http://www.glycemicindex.com/.

Chapter 22 – "Antioxidants and Supplements" Most of the information on the internet is slanted towards selling you something that is "rich in" or "loaded" with antioxidants and was the basis for including this chapter. You'll see that I use the term "may" throughout the chapter as there is very little conclusive evidence one way or the other on the benefit of antioxidants, especially if they are ingested in supplement form. The whole premise of this chapter is to help you to realize that if you eat a healthy diet, you won't have much to worry about when it comes to antioxidants and that there is no need to waste your money on worthless supplements. The recommendations for the three supplements worth considering (after consultation with your doctor) are my own.

The explanation of free radicals comes from "Understanding Free Radicals and Antioxidants" found on Health Check Systems at http://www.healthchecksystems.com/antioxid.htm. See also "Antioxidants and Fee Radicals" for and excellent article and a discussion of how infrequent exercise affects free radicals found at http://www.rice.edu/~jenky/sports/antiox.html.

There is mounting study evidence that we need more vitamin D, but recommendations on how we should get it is quite varied. I have tried to provide a consensus and like WebMD's "Vitamin D: Vital Role in Your Health at http://www.webmd.

com/food-recipes/features/vitamin-d-vital-role-in-your-health. Not only does this article have a great discussion on vitamin D, but it references all sorts of studies and is where I got my recommendation to get 5-10 minutes of sun on your bare arms and legs before you slather on the sunscreen.

The 2010 German study was widely reported in the press as you might expect when we hear it is good to eat (dark) chocolate. The actual study results were reprinted in the *European Heart Journal*, but you have to purchase the full text (abstract is free). Find it at: http://eurheartj.oxfordjournals.org/content/early/2010/03/18/eurheartj.ehq068.abstract.

Also see the International Osteoporosis Foundation's "New research clarifies roles of calcium, vitamin D, and protein in bone health, fracture risk" (Andrew Leopold) at: http://cmbi.bjmu.edu.cn/news/0606/30.htm for a good discussion of the value of vitamin D and dietary calcium. "Vitamin D and bone health in postmenopausal women" from the 12 March 2003 Journal or Women's Health (Malabanan AO & Holick MF) was also a useful resource. Find the abstract at: http://www.ncbi.nlm.nih.gov/pubmed/12737713.

The info on Eskimos came primarily from "How did Eskimos live for thousands of years on a diet of meat, seal, and fish without any of the vitamins and minerals in fruits and vegetables?" at http://www.answerbag.com/q_view/65929 and "Are you deficient? Too little vitamin D puts more than bones at risk," Nutrition Action Health Letter, Nov, 2006 by Bonnie Liebman found at: http://findarticles.com/p/articles/mi_m0813/is_9_33/ai_n16832548/.

There are dozens of omega-3 studies out there, and while there are still questions on whether or not we can all equally benefit from increased omega-3s, there is general consensus, that fish is better for you than cheeseburgers. If you are not a routine consumer of fish, it might make sense to ask your doctor about an omega-3 supplement. For and excellent synopsis of the benefits of omega-3s, see the Mayo Clinic's discussion on "omega-3 fatty acids, fish oil, alpha-linolenic acid available at http://www.mayoclinic.com/health/fish-oil/ ns_patient-fishoil/dsection=evidence.

Chapter 23 – "Label Reading 101" The FDA has taken some heat for not better defining or controlling what food manufacturers put on their food package labels, and their reluctance to define "100% Natural," "All Natural," or just plain "Natural" was widely reported in the press. A Mintel Market Survey in 2007 determined that "All natural" was the second most frequent claim on food labels. The first was "Kosher," with "No additives or preservatives" third. The definitions in this chapter (in italics) all come from the FDA web-site. Information on the specific foods mentioned come primarily from the company websites.

The FDA web-site does have some redeeming value and is a good resource for explanations of the Nutrition Facts Label and The Percent Daily Value (for key nutrients). See "How to Understand and Use the Nutrition Facts Label" at: http://www.fda.gov/Food/LabelingNutrition/ConsumerInformation/UCM078889.htm#nopercent.

The information on immunity boosting working for the elderly (defined as 65 and older) comes from a review of studies on nutritional intervention for older adults conducted by Dr. Kevin P. High of Wake Forest University School of Medicine in Winston-Salem, North Carolina. He found that the elderly can benefit from both mineral supplements and a daily multivitamin that helps to bring their daily intake of zinc, selenium and vitamin E to certain levels. The kicker is that Dr. High found evidence to suggest that "these supplements are likely to enhance immune function and may boost vaccine responses in healthy older adults." He also reported that supplements can help "Reduce the risk of infectious illness in both healthy and frail elders." This is a far cry from what is claimed on all the immunity boosting products out there today.

For a fuller and fascinating discussion on how we have come to define food almost solely based on sub-nutrients, read Michael Pollan's *"In Defense of Food, An Eater's Manifesto."* Once you have broken the code on weight loss, his instructions to "Eat food. Not too much. Mostly plants," will really resonate.

Chapter 24 – "It Costs $$ to Eat Well" is an acknowledgement that it costs a lot of money these days to eat the way you should. The genesis of this chapter was my wife's complaints and an article in my Tufts University Health & Nutrition Letter (from the Friedman School of Nutrition Science and Policy) titled "Can You Afford to Eat Right?" (May 2008).

The terms "energy dense" and "nutrient dense" come from this article, as do the quotes on the cost for both energy and nutrient rich diets. The information on how today's foods expertly combine salt, sugar and fats to make them almost impossible to resist comes from David Kessler's "The end of overeating."

The other Nutrition Newsletter I get each month is the "Nutrition Action Healthletter" published by the "Center For Science In The Public Interest." My Mom purchased a subscription for both my brother and me after our sister died and it is full of great advice each month. I especially like how they highlight their "Best Bites" each month, steering us towards foods that limit added sodium and fats. Subscribe at http://cspinet.org/nah/index.htm. There is a Canadian site as well.

Chapter 25 – "By The Numbers" All the FDA advice comes from their "How to understand and use the Nutrition Facts Label" available at: http://www.fda.gov/Food/LabelingNutrition/ConsumerInformation/UCM078889.htm. As stated in the text, my recommendations for losing weight are shown below the FDA advice and they are based on what is a reasonable goal to shoot for during a weight loss journey.

Chapter 26 –"Lose 30 Pounds in 30 Weeks" It seems to me that most people who check themselves against my Target Weight chart need to lose about 30 pounds, as I did. The lose 30 pounds in 30 weeks seems to be a goal that is well suited to the principles in this book. I also like keeping track of your weight each Friday so you can't kid yourself about the progress you're making. I actually kept my log in my *Day-Timer*, and encourage you to figure out a way to keep track of your progress. Once I realized I had it figured out and was making progress, it was thrilling to make a new, lower weight entry every Friday.

Chapter 27 – "Tying It All Together" is a compilation of everything I learned in the weight loss process. The idea for the Guiding Star came from Ida Halasz, PhD who has been an invaluable mentor, coach, editor and trusted advisor. Ida is also responsible for convincing me that "You Can't Outsource Weight Loss" (taken from a slide in my seminar PowerPoint) should really be the title of this book.

Lightning Source UK Ltd.
Milton Keynes UK
UKHW011833290322
400791UK00001B/27

9 780984 389803